ESSENTIALS of SURGICAL SPECIALTIES

ORAL EXAMINATIONS

ESSENTIALS of
SURGICAL SPECIALTIES
ORAL EXAMINATIONS

SENIOR EDITOR

Peter F. Lawrence, MD
Professor of Surgery
Department of Surgery
The University of Utah School of Medicine
Salt Lake City, Utah

EDITOR

Mitchell H. Goldman, MD
Professor of Surgery
Department of Surgery
University of Tennessee
    Medical Center at Knoxville
Knoxville, Tennessee

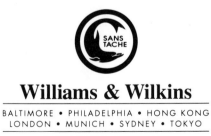

Williams & Wilkins
BALTIMORE • PHILADELPHIA • HONG KONG
LONDON • MUNICH • SYDNEY • TOKYO
A WAVERLY COMPANY

Editor: Timothy S. Satterfield
Managing Editor: Linda S. Napora
Copy Editor: Shelley Potler
Design: Norman W. Och
Production: Charles E. Zeller
Cover Designer: Michael Kotarba

Copyright © 1993
Williams & WIlkins
428 East Preston Street
Baltimore, Maryland 21202, USA

Accurate indications, adverse reactions, and dosage schedules for
drugs are provided in this book, but it is possible that they may
change. The reader is urged to review the package information data of
the manufacturers of the medications mentioned.

Printed in the United States of America

Library of Congress Cataloging-in-Publication Data

Oral examination questions to accompany Essentials of surgical
   specialties / senior editor, Peter F. Lawrence ; editor, Mitchell H.
   Goldman.
     p.   cm.
  Cover title: Essentials of surgical specialties, oral
examinations.
  ISBN 0-683-04865-1
   1. Surgery—Examinations, questions, etc. I. Lawrence, Peter F.
II. Goldman, Mitchell H. III. Essentials of surgical specialties.
IV. Title: Essentials of surgical specialties, oral examinations.
   [DNLM: 1. Surgery, Operative—examination questions. WO 500 E783
Suppl.]
RD31.E737 1993 Suppl.
617'.0076—dc20
DNLM/DLC
for Library of Congress   92-48675
                    CIP

93 94 95 96 97
1 2 3 4 5 6 7 8 9 10

To Margy, Mischa, Marshall, Matthew, and Meredith — the M&Ms

Preface

Essentials of Surgical Specialties is meant to serve as a complement to *Essentials of General Surgery*, which is oriented toward teaching what many feel is the information that all medical students need in general surgery by the end of their medical school career. *Essentials of Surgical Specialties* extends the information base into the surgical subspecialties.

Oral Examinations has been tailored to test the students' ability to put together factual information in a clinical situation to make correct diagnoses and institute appropriate therapies. Questions in *Oral Examinations* are completely based on the information in the textbook and were created by the authors of the individual chapters. It is our hope that, in the oral examination setting, the students will be tested on their ability to integrate the information in the textbook into clinical decision-making. The oral examination should be an opportunity for the student to demonstrate ability to solve problems in a clinical context. The oral examination setting should not be one in which the examiner's knowledge of trivia is the focus of the examination. Therefore, the questions have been standardized so that all examiners will be looking for similar information and show consistency in evaluation. Often, however, there are differences of opinion in surgical therapy and evaluation and as the questions are used, the examiners may wish to change different aspects of the questions. The questions are guides rather than absolutes. Embellishment, diversion from the main topic, and other directional changes that will bring out the student's fund of information are encouraged. Finally, the oral examination questions are in continuous flux and are subject to review, re-evaluation, and revision.

In the final analysis, it is the users who will decide whether the questions are worthwhile and it is our hope that you will give us the feedback necessary to make them so. With changing surgical information and philosophy, the book necessarily will need to evolve.

Although many have worked on this book, a note of great appreciation and thanks goes to Valerie Stamps for her hard work and help.

Contents

1 Anesthesiology

Case 1

A 10-year-old, 40-kg black male is scheduled for emergency appendectomy after presenting with a 2-day history of vomiting and fever. You are the anesthesia resident assigned to the case and see the child in the emergency room while he is being prepared for surgery.

OBJECTIVE 1

The student should obtain a history and conduct a physical examination before planning an anesthetic.
  A. Cardiovascular (no previous history of problems; heart examination normal except for rate of 140/minute).
  B. Respiratory (upper respiratory infection 1 week ago with no current cough or sore throat; lungs clear).
  C. Renal (no previous problems; no urine output since admission 2 hours ago).
  D. Metabolic (no history of any problems; temperature 104°F).
  E. Hematologic (family history of sickle cell disease; normal hemoglobin).
  F. Previous anesthetics (none).
  G. Family history of anesthetic problems (none).
  H. Current and previous medications and drug allergies (none).

OBJECTIVE 2

The student should evaluate the intravascular volume status.
  A. Intake over the past several hours (none).
  B. Blood pressure (BP) and heart rate (90/70 mm Hg, 140/minute).
  C. Skin turgor and appearance of mucosa (dry).
  D. Postural hypotension (BP falls to 70/40 mm Hg when patient sits up).
  E. Urine output (none in 2 hours).
  F. Resuscitation since admission (i.v. started in emergency room with 5% dextrose in lactated Ringer's solution [D_5LR] at 50 mL/hr).

OBJECTIVE 3

The student should determine whether the patient has a full stomach and is at risk for aspiration.
  A. Recent oral intake (none for 6 hours; no nasogastric tube in place).
  B. Vomiting (last episode 5 hours ago; clear liquid only).
  C. Peritonitis and bowel sounds (no bowel sounds).

OBJECTIVE 4

The student should determine what laboratory tests are needed.
  A. Complete blood count (CBC — hemoglobin [Hb] 10.9 g/dL, hematocrit [Hct] 40%, white blood cells [WBC] 15,000/mm^3 with a left shift).
  B. Electrolytes (Na$^+$ 150, K$^+$ 3.0, Cl$^-$ 120, HCO$_3^-$ 16).
  C. Other tests (blood urea nitrogen [BUN] 23 mg/dL, chest x-ray normal).

OBJECTIVE 5

The student should prepare the patient for anesthesia.
  A. Prepare patient psychologically and obtain informed consent (reassure patient; obtain parents' agreement for general anesthesia).
  B. Ensure adequacy of i.v. (18-gauge catheter running well).
  C. Determine preoperative medication (no sedatives or narcotics because of reduced blood volume status; H$_2$-blockers will not work fast enough to protect against aspiration pneumonitis).
  D. Outline monitoring plan (routine monitors required; no central venous pressure (CVP) since patient's condition is good and blood volume status assessed by vital signs and urine output; needs Foley catheter).
  E. Administer fluid bolus and prepare to replace potassium intraoperatively with ECG monitoring (patient is hypovolemic, acidotic, hypokalemic, needs further fluid resuscitation).

F. Plan induction and maintenance based on patient's medical status and surgeon's requirements (possible full stomach; general anesthesia with rapid sequence induction or awake intubation; some muscle relaxation needed; patient does not want spinal or epidural anesthetic).

Additional Questions

1. What risk does dehydration present for this patient?
2. Would a spinal anesthetic be safer for this patient?

Achievement Level

OBJECTIVE 1

Minimum Level of Achievement for Passing

The student should:

A. Obtain a history of cardiac, respiratory, renal, and metabolic problems.
B. Ask about the respiratory infection, determining if there was fever, cough, antibiotic medication, and how long the patient has been free of symptoms.
C. Listen to the heart and lungs and ensure that a chest x-ray has been obtained.
D. Question the parents about the patient's previous anesthetics, medications, and allergies.

Honors Level of Achievement

The student should:

A. Ask whether the patient has ever been tested for sickle cell disease.
B. Ask about family history of anesthesia problems, looking for inherited malignant hyperthermia and porphyrias.

OBJECTIVE 2

Minimum Level of Achievement for Passing

The student should:

A. Be aware the patient is severely dehydrated because of acute disease, BP, and tachycardia.
B. Ask about urine output and amount of i.v. fluid administered.
C. Be able to assess blood volume status by examining the patient's skin and mucous membranes.

Honors Level of Achievement

The student should check for postural hypotension.

OBJECTIVE 3

Minimum Level of Achievement for Passing

The student should:

A. Consider the possibility of a full stomach and the risk for aspiration pneumonitis in any emergency surgery.

B. Consider the risk even though the patient has been vomiting.

Honors Level of Achievement

The student should know the stomach may be full whenever there is intraperitoneal pathology that could decrease gastrointestinal (GI) motility.

OBJECTIVE 4

Minimum Level of Achievement for Passing

The student should:

A. Ask for a CBC, electrolytes, and BUN.
B. Anticipate that Hct and Na^+ will be high, and that K^+ and HCO_3^- be low.

Honors Level of Achievement

The student should discuss the implications of electrolyte abnormalities and formulate a plan for correcting them intraoperatively.

OBJECTIVE 5

Minimum Level of Achievement for Passing

The student should:

A. Be able to discuss possible anesthetic techniques with the patient and parents.
B. Understand that a large-bore, well-functioning i.v. line must be in place and that further fluid resuscitation is necessary before inducing anesthesia.
C. Discuss aspiration prevention by awake or rapid sequence induction.
D. List the routine monitors required for every anesthetic: BP, ECG, stethoscope, pulse oximeter, capnograph, temperature.

Honors Level of Achievement

The student should:

A. Discuss methods of assessing blood volume status intraoperatively, including BP, heart rate, urine output, and pulse characteristics.
B. Discuss the indications for CVP monitoring.

Additional Questions

Minimum Level of Achievement for Passing

The student should:

A. Be aware that reduced circulating blood volume results in hypotension when vasodilating anesthetic agents are administered for induction and maintenance of anesthesia.
B. Be aware that suppression of autonomic activity during anesthesia contributes to hypotension.
C. Be aware that blood and insensible fluid loss and fluid sequestration in the postoperative period will require monitoring of volume status.
D. Know that if the spinal anesthetic were free of complications it would eliminate the risk of

aspiration pneumonitis but might cause a greater degree of hypotension.

E. Know that the patient, frightened of a needle puncture, would probably be difficult to manage during a spinal anesthetic.

Honors Level of Achievement

The student should:

A. Know that because dehydrated patients are at risk for developing oliguria, kidney function should be monitored using frequent determinations of urine output.

B. Know that there is no evidence that the patient would have a better outcome with either a spinal or a regional anesthetic.

Case 2

You are an anesthesia resident making preoperative rounds. A 65-year-old male with angina and claudication needs a right femoral-popliteal bypass. The admitting ECG shows evidence of an old anterolateral myocardial infarction and a left bundle branch block. How do you prepare this patient for anesthesia and surgery?

OBJECTIVE 1

The student should obtain a history, physical examination, and laboratory data.

A. Cardiac status (history of dyspnea and angina on exertion; recent activity severely limited by claudication; no orthopnea; no angina at rest; no medications).

B. Vascular status (no carotid bruits; peripheral pulses absent in right foot but otherwise all right).

C. Renal status (BUN and creatinine normal).

OBJECTIVE 2

Knowing that there are new ECG changes and symptomatic myocardial ischemic episodes as well as untreated hypertension, the student should formulate a plan for a comprehensive cardiovascular workup and BP control before surgery.

A. Ask the patient's primary care physician or a cardiologist to help optimize BP control and assess the status of myocardial perfusion.

B. Obtain a series of BP measurements to determine the range.

C. Consult the anesthesiologist involved, so that he or she can participate in the patient's preparation and begin planning the intraoperative management.

OBJECTIVE 3

The student should determine when the patient is in optimum condition for surgery.

A. Control BP through a stable medication regimen.

B. Assess the state of myocardial contractility, using echocardiography or further tests of myocardial function; optimize by medication if necessary.

C. Assess the degree of myocardial ischemia and whether dipyridamole-thallium scanning may be required; understand the conditions that bring it on.

D. Control any preventable or reversible ischemia using medications, angioplasty, or even coronary artery bypass surgery if necessary.

OBJECTIVE 4

The student should indicate the monitors that may be used perioperatively to ensure optimal myocardial protection and organ perfusion.

A. Monitors of myocardial perfusion (ECG, S-T segment trending, transesophageal echocardiography).

B. Monitors of volume status (CVP, pulmonary artery and wedge pressures, cardiac outputs, mixed venous oxygen saturations, noninvasive and invasive blood pressure determination, urine output, pulse oximetry).

Additional Questions

The patient has been stabilized on nitropaste, a β-blocker, and a diuretic. His BP values have been in the range of 120–140/80–90 mm Hg for a few days. He has a fixed regional wall motion abnormality and a good ejection fraction on echocardiography; he has had no other testing.

1. Is he ready?
2. Should he have invasive monitoring?
3. What anesthetic should be chosen?

Achievement Level

OBJECTIVE 1

Minimum Level of Achievement for Passing

The student should:

A. Obtain a history from the patient that includes the degree and frequency of angina, past medications, and signs and symptoms of congestive heart failure.

B. Suspect other vascular disease and look for signs and symptoms of carotid, renal, and aortic insufficiency.

Honors Level of Achievement

The student should:

A. Indicate the chest x-ray gives important information in the workup of heart disease.

B. Should understand the importance of obtaining previous ECG tracings for comparison.

OBJECTIVE 2

Minimum Level of Achievement for Passing

The student should:

A. Consider the primary care physician's information in determining the status of the patient's cardiovascular system and in stabilizing him.

B. Be aware of the benefits of early consultation with the anesthesiologist.

C. Be aware that one single BP determination is inadequate in diagnosing hypertension.

Honors Level of Achievement

The student should discuss the expertise a cardiologist brings to the situation, including invasive techniques to assess and optimize myocardial oxygenation.

OBJECTIVE 3

Minimum Level of Achievement for Passing

The student should:

A. Require that BP readings be stabilized on medication within a certain range for at least a day.

B. Discuss the information obtained from echocardiography, including wall motion and left ventricular ejection fraction, and the information obtained from a dipyridamole-thallium scan.

C. Suggest medications that optimize myocardial performance, including digitalis preparations and coronary vasodilators.

Honors Level of Achievement

The student should explain under what conditions surgery should be postponed until angioplasty or revascularization is accomplished.

OBJECTIVE 4

Minimum Level of Achievement for Passing

The student should:

A. Discuss what information can be gathered from each monitor.

B. Indicate the situations where intraarterial pressure monitoring is desirable.

Honors Level of Achievement

The student should be able to give examples of specific conditions where pulmonary artery catheters are indicated, such as for low left ventricular ejection fractions or cardiac output determinations.

Additional Questions

Minimum Level of Achievement for Passing

The student should:

A. Know to proceed with the surgery with the medications continued throughout the perioperative period.

B. Choose to use intraarterial pressure monitoring (because of possible rapid swings in BP) and central pressure monitoring (to anticipate problems in maintaining intravascular volume without overloading the heart).

C. Know that the choice of anesthetic technique is optional, depending on the preferences of the patient, the surgeon, and the anesthesiologist.

Honors Level of Achievement

The student should discuss the situations in which a pulmonary artery catheter is preferable to a right atrial pressure monitor during surgery. The student should note that if left ventricular ejection fraction is 40% or less, right heart pressures do not always reflect circulating volume.

Case 3

The ophthalmologist scheduling a 65-year-old diabetic patient for outpatient cataract removal under monitored anesthesia care calls you, the resident, in the preanesthesia clinic. How should you prepare the patient?

OBJECTIVE 1

The student should indicate that the anesthesiologist's evaluation should be performed as early as possible, preferably a few days before the surgery, and include careful assessment of:

A. Diabetes
1. Medication (oral hypoglycemics once daily, diet control).
2. Compliance (patient checks urine daily, rarely spills glucose).
3. Nutritional status (patient is obese: weight 100 kg, height 5'8").
4. Glucose (random glucose 240 mg/dL, urine glucose and ketones negative).
5. Other (no history of neuropathy; electrolytes, BUN, and creatinine normal).

B. Cardiovascular system (BP 140/85 mm Hg, rate 80/minute; no history of angina, congestive failure, dyspnea; ECG — frequent unifocal premature ventricular contractions (PVCs), otherwise normal).

C. Respiratory system (examination and chest x-ray normal).

OBJECTIVE 2

The student should explain how the patient is prepared for surgery.

A. The surgeon should discuss local anesthetic and procedure, and obtain informed consent.

B. The anesthesiologist should describe the operating room, monitors, intravenous fluids, sedation that will be used, and obtain informed consent.

C. The patient should be instructed to remain n.p.o. (nothing by mouth) after midnight, not to take hypoglycemic medication before arriving at the hospital, and to arrive in time to allow a preoperative examination and glucose determination.

D. The patient should be prepared for possible postoperative hospitalization to control diabetes.

OBJECTIVE 3

The student should describe immediate preoperative preparation.

A. Dextrose-containing solution administered i.v.; blood drawn for glucose determination (if glucose high, insulin should be administered and repeat determinations done every hour).

B. Heart and lungs reexamined; patient questioned again about oral intake.

C. ECG applied before local anesthesia is injected; patient monitored continuously throughout injection and after.

D. Oxygen administered through nasal cannula.

E. Operating room monitoring to include ECG, BP every 5 minutes, precordial stethoscope for breath and heart sounds, pulse oximetry, frequent verbal contact.

OBJECTIVE 4

The student should discuss appropriate intravenous sedation, which may include small doses of any short-acting narcotics and/or sedatives.

OBJECTIVE 5

The student should discuss the complications of local anesthetics.

A. Drug toxicity (CNS, cardiac).

B. Intravascular injection (seizures; treatment — O_2, ventilation if necessary, anticonvulsants, muscle relaxants).

C. Allergic reactions.

OBJECTIVE 6

The student should be aware of indications for postoperative hospitalization.

A. Pain requiring narcotic injections.

B. Intractable nausea and/or vomiting precluding oral intake.

C. Severe hyperglycemia requiring insulin therapy.

D. Surgical or anesthetic complications.

E. Continued sedation precluding ambulation.

Additional Questions

The patient is a type I diabetic on 40 units of NPH insulin in the morning and 20 units in the evening. How do you manage the diabetes in this situation?

Achievement Level

OBJECTIVE 1

Minimum Level of Achievement for Passing

The student should:

A. Know that the anesthesiologist should see the patient as soon as possible, so that further workup can be arranged if necessary.

B. Be alert to the possibility of cardiovascular, renal, and neurologic problems concurrent with diabetes.

C. Be aware of the patient's degree of diabetic control and institute better control if necessary.

D. Know that the minimal laboratory workup must include CBC, electrolytes, kidney function, ECG, and chest x-ray.

Honors Level of Achievement

The student should determine whether the patient has any discomfort, airway obstruction, or dyspnea in the supine position.

OBJECTIVE 2

Minimum Level of Achievement for Passing

The student should:

A. Allay the patient's fears about the surgical procedure and about being awake in the operating room.

B. Describe to the patient the medication to be administered on the day of surgery and the importance of presenting with an empty stomach.

Honors Level of Achievement

The student should present an argument that would persuade a reluctant patient to allow surgery under local anesthesia.

OBJECTIVE 3

Minimal Level of Achievement for Passing

The student should:

A. Discuss the perioperative control of glucose in the diabetic patient, including glucose administration, laboratory testing, and sliding scale insulin therapy.

B. Understand the necessity of monitoring the patient during and after injection of the local anesthetic around the eye.

C. Describe the minimal monitoring necessary during the procedure.

Honors Level of Achievement

The student should anticipate the need for supplementary oxygen administration (because the patient's face is draped and because of the effects of sedation).

OBJECTIVE 4

Minimum Level of Achievement for Passing

The student should know the types of drugs that are used for supplementary intravenous sedation, and the need for careful titration of small doses.

Honors Level of Achievement

The student should describe the doses, side effects, and duration of action of fentanyl, midazolam, Valium, and droperidol when used in this setting.

OBJECTIVE 5

Minimum Level of Achievement for Passing

The student should:
  A. Discuss the signs of impending CNS toxicity (shivering, jitteriness, ringing in the ears, circumoral numbness).
  B. Discuss the treatment of seizures and list oxygen as the first treatment.
  C. Know the cardiovascular effects of local anesthetics, and that the only treatment is prolonged resuscitation or support.

Honors Level of Achievement

The student should know that in cases of high blood levels of local anesthetics, it is difficult to distinguish between allergic reactions and toxic effects.

OBJECTIVE 6

Minimum Level of Achievement for Passing

The student should be aware of the listed indications for this patient's hospitalization.

Honors Level of Achievement

The student should describe the treatment of nausea in the immediate postoperative period, and should list methods of pain relief acceptable in the ambulatory patient.

Additional Question

Minimum Level of Achievement for Passing

The student should:
  A. Outline patient preparations to be taken the night before surgery (the patient should take her insulin, keep a glass of juice by her bed, and come to the hospital early the next day).
  B. Outline patient management on admission (a glucose i.v. should be started and half the usual dose of NPH given).
  C. Outline patient monitoring during surgery (glucose determinations should be made hourly and additional regular insulin given as needed — tight or loose control, as desired).
  D. Outline criteria patient should meet before discharge (patient should be able to take p.o. (by mouth) liquids, is not excessively hyperglycemic or ketotic, and is able to take over her own control).

Honors Level of Achievement

The student should be able to outline an alternate plan, resulting in tight control, which would consist of starting simultaneous i.v. lines of D_5 and insulin; the plan's adequacy should be checked by hourly glucose determinations.

Case 4

Your otherwise normal patient is in the recovery room after undergoing an uneventful thyroidectomy under general anesthesia with fentanyl, isoflurane, and N_2O. She suddenly becomes agitated and hypertensive. As the anesthesia resident in the recovery room, what do you do?

OBJECTIVE 1

The student should generate a differential diagnosis of postoperative excitement and hypertension. This should include hypoxia, pain, respiratory insufficiency, acidosis, emergence delirium, hypothermia, hypervolemia, shock, naloxone.

OBJECTIVE 2

The student should suggest immediate steps to be taken to evaluate the cause.
  A. Examination (heart rate 140/minute; BP 160/100 mm Hg; auscultation of the heart and lungs — no abnormal findings except rapid 40/minute shallow respirations; pupils dilated; no hematoma visible on neck; patient complaining of pain and nausea).
  B. Monitors (ECG shows only tachycardia; pulse oximeter SaO_2 96% on 40% O_2; temperature 96°F axillary).
  C. Laboratory evaluation (blood gas analysis pH 7.45, $PaCO_2$ 35 mm Hg, PaO_2 90 mm Hg, Hct 30%).

OBJECTIVE 3

The student should present a defensible assessment of the problem.
  A. No previous history of hypertension.
  B. Patient neither hypoxic nor hypoventilating; no sign of upper airway obstruction from surgery.
  C. Residual anesthetic effects not apparent (pupils, respiratory pattern, complaints of pain indicate no residual narcotization).

D. Diagnosis (pain and/or emergence excitement).

OBJECTIVE 4

The student should generate a reasonable plan.
   A. After an initial dose, the patient should be given small incremental doses of narcotic, either in i.v. boluses or, preferably, with patient-controlled analgesia (PCA).
   B. Nausea should be treated with prochlorperazine, droperidol, or similar drug.

OBJECTIVE 5

The student should demonstrate the ability to assess the results of therapy.
   A. Patient response (10 minutes after i.v. morphine, 5 mg, and droperidol, 1.25 mg, the patient is quieter).
   B. Vital signs (respiratory rate 12/minute, heart rate 100/minute, BP 140/80 mm Hg, SaO_2 98%).

Additional Questions

1. The patient was not agitated but was hypertensive and tachycardic. On initial assessment she had a respiratory rate of 6/minute, a $PaCO_2$ of 60 mm Hg, and her pupils were pinpoint. What is the most likely diagnosis and treatment?
2. After receiving morphine, 5 mg, and droperidol, 1.25 mg i.v., the patient becomes calmer but the hypertension persists. What do you do now?

Achievement Level

OBJECTIVE 1

Minimum Level of Achievement for Passing

The student's differential diagnosis should include all of the listed possibilities.

Honors Level of Achievement

The student's differential diagnosis should begin with hypoxia.

OBJECTIVE 2

Minimum Level of Achievement for Passing

The student should:
   A. Assess the heart rate and rhythm, BP, ECG, and respiratory pattern; auscultate the heart and lungs.
   B. Assess the patient's mental status.
   C. Ask about the patient's SaO_2 and temperature.
   D. Obtain blood gases before treating the patient with narcotics.

Honors Level of Achievement

The student should:
   A. Remember that because the surgery was on the neck, there is a potential for upper airway obstruction from hematoma or swelling.
   B. Check the pupils for signs of residual narcotization.
   C. Obtain blood gases before treating the patient with narcotics.

OBJECTIVE 3

Minimum Level of Achievement for Passing

The student should conclude that pain is the most probable cause, after determining that the patient is not hypoxic or in respiratory distress.

Honors Level of Achievement

In coming to this conclusion, the student should also note the absence of previous history of hypertension.

OBJECTIVE 4

Minimum Level of Achievement for Passing

The student should present a plan for treating the pain and nausea.

Honors Level of Achievement

The student should mention PCA and the drugs and doses for antiemetics.

OBJECTIVE 5

Minimum Level of Achievement for Passing

The student should list criteria for establishing that the treatment is adequate.

Honors Level of Achievement

Should the treatment not be adequate, the student should have a plan of action, such as further titration of drugs or reassessment of the patient.

Additional Questions

Minimum Level of Achievement for Passing

The student should:
   A. Recognize signs of residual narcotization, which causes hypoventilation.
   B. Be aware that hypertension and tachycardia are most likely due to sympathetic stimulation from hypercarbia.
   C. Outline a plan of action to support respiration until the narcotic wears off, or to administer small incremental doses of naloxone to reverse the respiratory depression but still preserve the analgesia.
   D. Consider treating hypertension with appropriately titrated i.v. doses of a rapid-acting antihypertensive such as propranolol, esmolol, labetalol, or hydralazine.

E. Demonstrate that he would first insert an arterial line for continuous monitoring before using a continuous i.v. drip of a potent vasodilator such as nitroprusside.

Honors Level of Achievement

The student should:
A. Know how to administer naloxone in this situation and be aware of its possible side effects (it should be titrated carefully after first assisting the patient's ventilation to reduce hypercarbia; side effects include further sympathetic stimulation — resulting in severe hypertension and tachycardia that may progress to pulmonary edema — and seizures.
B. Be able to discuss the relative merits of β-blocking agents and vasodilators in this situation.

Case 5

During general anesthesia, which you are administering for a hepatic tumor resection in an otherwise normal young adult, the BP reading from an arterial line gradually (over 5 minutes) falls from 100/80 mm Hg to 70/30 mm Hg. Other monitors in place include CVP, Foley catheter, pulse oximeter, capnograph, oxygen analyzer, and temperature probe.

OBJECTIVE 1

The student should immediately check information from all of the other monitors.
A. ECG (heart rate 140/minute, rhythm regular, complexes unchanged from previous).
B. Arterial line tracing (slow upsweep, marked variation in pressure with respirations).
C. Volume status (CVP, 0 to 1; urine output in last half-hour, 10 mL).
D. Pulse oximeter (not detecting a pulse in the finger).
E. Oxygen analyzer (expired O_2 reading 50%).
F. Capnograph (has fallen from 35 mm Hg to 20 mm Hg).
G. Temperature (unchanged from 35°C).

OBJECTIVE 2

The student should examine the patient.
A. Skin (pale, dry, poor capillary refill).
B. Heart sounds (distant).
C. Breath sounds (unchanged).
D. Peripheral pulses (thready, barely palpable).
E. Pupils (small, nonreactive).

OBJECTIVE 3

The student should rapidly assess the situation to determine the most likely cause: sudden blood loss, anesthetic overdose, inadequate volume replacement, circulatory collapse.
A. Blood loss (the surgical field, suction, and sponges indicate total blood loss of about 1000 mL since the beginning of the procedure; no blood has been given).
B. Anesthetic (nothing has changed recently; the vaporizer setting and gas flows are the same; no recent narcotics or sedatives have been administered).
C. Circulating blood volume (total of 1000 mL lactated Ringer's solution has been given; surgery has been proceeding for 2 hours; CVP and urine output very low; pulse tracing indicates a cardiac output that varies markedly with respiration; pulse oximeter and palpation of the peripheral pulses indicate hypovolemia; sudden fall in expired CO_2 provides further evidence of decreased cardiac output).
D. Cardiovascular collapse (ECG complexes unchanged; myocardial ischemia not profound enough to affect cardiac output).

OBJECTIVE 4

The student should generate a plan for immediate action.
A. Volume infusion (determine patient's Hct before transfusing blood; infuse crystalloid or colloid solution).
B. Inhaled anesthetic administration (decrease concentration until BP is stabilized).
C. Drugs (consider only if rapid volume infusion and decreasing anesthetic concentration do not help soon; myocardium and brain being perfused adequately).

OBJECTIVE 5

The student should be able to assess the results of initial therapy and plan further action accordingly.
A. After infusing 500 mL crystalloid and decreasing inspired anesthetic concentration, BP stabilizes at 100/60 mm Hg, pulse 100/minute; pulse oximeter reads 100% saturation, and capnograph reads 30 mm Hg.
B. Hct drawn at the time of the hypotensive episode is 25%; patient should begin receiving blood transfusion, and further blood loss replaced promptly.
C. Fluid infusion for the rest of the procedure should proceed at a faster rate.
D. Depth of anesthesia should be reassessed to determine optimal level.

Additional Questions

1. In the above situation, BP was 70/30 mm Hg, heart rate was 40/minute, CVP was 15; urine output was not decreased, ECG complexes were unchanged, and expired CO_2 and O_2 were also unchanged from before the hypotension. What is the most likely diagnosis and treatment?
2. During major abdominal surgery such as this, when is the insertion of a pulmonary arterial catheter indicated?

Achievement Level

OBJECTIVE 1

Minimum Level of Achievement for Passing

The student should:
A. Immediately check information from the other monitors to assess the cause of hypotension.
B. Ask about the pulse rate first, then about the ECG, pulse oximeter, expired O_2, and respiratory monitors.
C. Ask for a CVP reading and what the urine output has been.

Honors Level of Achievement

The student should be able to discuss the causes of a sudden fall in expired CO_2 and indicate that a decrease in cardiac output is among those causes.

OBJECTIVE 2

Minimum Level of Achievement for Passing

The student should rapidly assess the patient for signs of decreased peripheral perfusion and for adequacy of respiration and heart sounds.

Honors Level of Achievement

The student should check the pupils for signs of brain hypoxia.

OBJECTIVE 3

Minimum Level of Achievement for Passing

The student should:
A. Make a provisional diagnosis of hypovolemia, either from blood loss or from inadequate volume infusion during surgery.
B. Consider the probability that vasodilating effects of the inhaled anesthetic are contributing to the problem.
C. Not suspect myocardial dysfunction because of normal ECG and low CVP.

Honors Level of Achievement

The student should:
A. Check blood loss first.

B. Consider possibility of anesthetic overdose only secondarily, given the nature of the surgery.
C. State the infusion rate of crystalloid required to replace insensible loss during major abdominal surgery.

OBJECTIVE 4

Minimum Level of Achievement for Passing

The student should:
A. Begin treatment with rapid infusion of crystalloid and obtain an Hct to decide whether to transfuse blood.
B. Understand that because inhaled anesthetic contributes to hypotension, its concentration should be reduced until BP returns to a more acceptable level.

Honors Level of Achievement

The student should not administer vasoconstrictors for hypovolemia unless there is evidence of brain or myocardial ischemia.

Additional Questions

Minimum Level of Achievement for Passing

The student should:
A. Recognize cardiovascular depression caused by the depressant effects of the anesthetic.
B. Outline treatment consisting of discontinuing the inhalational agent, watching monitors to see if the depression begins to reverse, and administering supportive drugs and continuing investigation into its causes if it does not.
C. Know to insert a pulmonary arterial catheter when (a) the patient's circulating volume cannot be accurately assessed with a CVP and a Foley catheter and (b) when the patient's medical condition and the surgery will likely require cardiac output determinations, mixed venous oxygen saturation determinations, or the possibility of pacing — as when a patient is in septic shock.

Honors Level of Achievement

The student should:
A. Discuss the advantages and disadvantages of dopamine, dobutamine, amrinone, epinephrine, and isoproterenol in this situation.
B. Give examples of when a patient is likely to need a pulmonary arterial catheter (when there is right heart failure, pulmonary hypertension, or when in left ventricular failure there is an ejection fraction of less than 40%).

2 Pediatric Surgery: Surgical Diseases of Children

Case 1

A 5-year-old girl presents with a 36-hour history of right lower quadrant pain becoming generalized, with bilious vomiting and fever.

OBJECTIVE 1

The student should elicit further history from the child and her parents.
  A. Pain (started around the belly button).
  B. Appetite (anorexic for 24 hours).
  C. Symptoms (parents thought she had the flu).
  D. Last void (parents cannot remember when she last voided).
  E. Previous illness (she has not been sick like this in the past).

OBJECTIVE 2

The student should perform an appropriate physical examination.
  A. General (ill-appearing child with dry mucous membranes; child not moving).
  B. Vital signs (tympanic temperature, 39°C; weight, 20 kg; pulse, 150/min; respiratory rate, 40/min; blood pressure [BP], 100/60 mm Hg).
  C. Chest (splinting, decreased breath sounds at bases, heart sounds normal).
  D. Abdomen (distended, rigid, generalized percussion tenderness).
  E. Rectum (tender above peritoneal reflection).

OBJECTIVE 3

The student should diagnose a surgical abdomen, probable perforated appendicitis, and order appropriate laboratory and x-ray studies.
  A. Complete blood count (CBC) (white blood cells [WBC] 17,500/mm³, neutrophils [neuts] 75%, bands 20%, lymphs 5%, hematocrit [Hct] 42%, hemoglobin [Hgb] 14 g/dL, platelets 150,000/mm³).

  B. Urinalysis (ketones 3+, specific gravity [sp gr] 1.029, microscopic negative).
  C. Electrolytes (sodium [Na] 137 mEq/L, potassium [K] 4.3 mEq/L).
  D. Chest x-ray (lung fields clear, diaphragms elevated).
  E. Abdominal x-ray (dilated small and large bowel, air in rectum, no free air).

OBJECTIVE 4

The student should outline preoperative preparations.
  A. Start i.v.: bolus of 200–400 mL lactated Ringer's, then run at 200–400 mL/hr until hydrated.
  B. Administer triple i.v. antibiotics: gentamicin, ampicillin, and clindamycin.
  C. Insert nasogastric sump and place to suction.
  D. Administer rectal Tylenol to decrease temperature and anesthetic risk (optional).
  E. Obtain informed operative consent from parents, telling them diagnosis cannot be 100% certain; the risks involved include wound or intraabdominal infection and adhesions.
  F. Tell child she will sleep while you make her tummy better, her parents will be with her when she wakes up, and she may have a nose tube when she wakes up.

Achievement Level

OBJECTIVE 1

Minimum Level of Achievement for Passing

The student should:
  A. Obtain history from patient and accompanying adults.
  B. Elicit pain progression.
  C. Perform gastrointestinal review of symptoms.

Honors Level of Achievement

The student should:
  A. Ask time of last void, and concentration if known.

B. Already be considering the possibility of appendicitis.

OBJECTIVE 2

Minimum Level of Achievement for Passing

The student should:
A. Make a visual assessment of the child, including movement.
B. Obtain vital signs and weight.
C. Perform complete abdominal examination, in correct order.

Honors Level of Achievement

The student should:
A. Know which vital signs are abnormal values for age.
B. Perform a rectal examination.

OBJECTIVE 3

Minimum Level of Achievement for Passing

The student should:
A. Make a diagnosis of surgical abdomen, probable appendicitis.
B. Order CBC, urinalysis, electrolytes, and x-rays.
C. Recognize dehydration and leukocytosis with left shift.

Honors Level of Achievement

The student should:
A. Make diagnosis of perforated appendix.
B. Be able to explain presence of ketones in urine.

OBJECTIVE 4

Minimum Level of Achievement for Passing

The student should:
A. Immediately start 10–20 mL/kg lactated Ringer's bolus.
B. Order antibiotics effective against enteric organisms.
C. Establish continuous nasogastric decompression.

Honors Level of Achievement

The student should:
A. Communicate with child and parents.
B. Know complications of perforated appendix.

Case 2

A 4-year-old girl presents with bilious vomiting, cramping abdominal pain, chills, and fever.

OBJECTIVE 1

The student should elicit further history from the child and her parents.
A. Other symptoms (cough 2 days ago was treated with Dimetapp).
B. Appetite (became anorectic yesterday).
C. Stool (normal yesterday).
D. Last void (7 hours ago).
E. Previous hospitalization or surgery (none).

OBJECTIVE 2

The student should perform an appropriate physical examination.
A. General (tachypneic child with nasal flaring).
B. Vital signs (tympanic temperature, 39.8°C; weight, 18 kg; pulse, 164/minute; respiratory rate, 80/minute).
C. Head, eyes, ears, nose, throat (normal).
D. Chest (lungs clear to auscultation but too dry for rales, heart regular without murmur).
E. Abdomen (bowel sounds decreased, rigid and diffusely tender to light palpation, especially around the umbilicus).

OBJECTIVE 3

The student should order and interpret appropriate laboratory and x-ray studies.
A. CBC (WBC 37,000/mm^3, neuts 74%, bands 22%, lymphs 4%, Hgb 15 g/dL, Hct 45%, platelets 350,000/mm^3).
B. Urinalysis (ketones 3+, sp gr 1.027, dipstick negative).
C. Electrolytes (normal, not essential).
D. Chest x-ray (left lower lobe pneumonia, best seen on lateral view).
E. Abdominal x-ray (mild dilation of small and large intestine with scattered air-fluid levels, air in rectum).

OBJECTIVE 4

The student should make a diagnosis of left lower lobe pneumonia and discuss further appropriate management.
A. Admit to the hospital.
B. Draw blood cultures (patient this age will not produce sputum for culture).
C. Start i.v. of lactated Ringer's at 180–360 mL/hr.
D. Administer i.v. antibiotics covering community-acquired respiratory organisms, including *Haemophilus*.
E. Physical examination changes (rales appear with hydration).

Achievement Level

OBJECTIVE 1

Minimum Level of Achievement for Passing

The student should:
  A. Obtain history from patient and accompanying adults.
  B. Elicit history of cough.
  C. Perform gastrointestinal review of symptoms.

Honors Level of Achievement

The student should
  A. Ask time of last void, and concentration if known.
  B. Suspect appendicitis.

OBJECTIVE 2

Minimum Level of Achievement for Passing

The student should:
  A. Recognize increased respiratory effort.
  B. Obtain vital signs and weight.
  C. Examine chest and abdomen thoroughly.

Honors Level of Achievement

The student should:
  A. Recognize that respiratory rate and nasal flaring are inconsistent with an intraabdominal process.
  B. Know that fever is very high for appendicitis.

OBJECTIVE 3

Minimum Level of Achievement for Passing

The student should:
  A. Order CBC, urinalysis, chest and abdominal films.
  B. Recognize leukocytosis and dehydration.
  C. Read chest x-ray appropriately.

Honors Level of Achievement

The student should:
  A. Recognize that WBC is very high for appendicitis.
  B. Identify ileus from diaphragmatic irritation.

OBJECTIVE 4

Minimum Level of Achievement for Passing

The student should:
  A. Diagnose pneumonia and admit patient.
  B. Start i.v. fluids above maintenance rate.
  C. Order antibiotics for community-acquired pneumonia.

Honors Level of Achievement

The student should:
  A. Recognize that child is too young to produce sputum.
  B. Realize that child is too dehydrated to have rales.

Case 3

A 3-month-old boy is brought to clinic because his parents have noticed a painless, intermittent right inguinal and scrotal swelling for 3 days. He is taking antibiotics for treatment of otitis media.

OBJECTIVE 1

The student should elicit further history from the parents.
  A. Swelling (largest when infant is crying or straining to stool; not present when infant is sleeping).
  B. Constipation (none).
  C. Birth (infant born at term without neonatal problems).
  D. Immunizations (current).

OBJECTIVE 2

The student should perform an appropriate physical examination.
  A. General (vigorous, active infant).
  B. Vital signs (tympanic temperature, 37.3°C; weight, 5 kg; pulse, 140/minute; respiratory rate, 30/minute).
  C. Head, eyes, ears, nose, throat (nasal crusting, right tympanic membrane red and bulging without light reflex).
  D. Chest (coarse upper airway sounds, heart regular without murmur).
  E. Abdomen (soft without palpable mass).
  F. Genital examination (no inguinal or scrotal swelling on initial examination; crying produces easily reducible right inguinal and scrotal bulge).

OBJECTIVE 3

The student should diagnose an inguinal hernia and describe appropriate management.
  A. High risk for incarceration.
  B. Significant incidence of bilaterality.
  C. Outpatient surgery.
  D. Schedule repair 2 weeks after upper respiratory infection (URI) resolves.
  E. Right inguinal hernia repair with left inguinal exploration.

Achievement Level

OBJECTIVE 1

Minimum Level of Achievement for Passing

The student should:
  A. Obtain history from infant's parents.
  B. Elicit relationship of swelling to activity.
  C. Acquire birth and immunization history.

Honors Level of Achievement

The student should:
  A. Ask about predisposing conditions.
  B. Already be considering the possibility of inguinal hernia.

OBJECTIVE 2

Minimum Level of Achievement for Passing

The student should:
  A. Recognize signs of URI.
  B. Obtain vital signs and weight.
  C. Stimulate infant to cry to reproduce bulge.

Honors Level of Achievement

The student should:
  A. Realize that URI increases intraabdominal pressure.
  B. Be able to describe pediatric groin examination.

OBJECTIVE 3

Minimum Level of Achievement for Passing

The student should:
  A. Diagnose inguinal hernia.
  B. Refer infant for outpatient repair.
  C. Know that there is a significant risk of incarceration in infant.

Honors Level of Achievement

The student should:
  A. Know that the incidence of bilaterality is high.
  B. Realize that repair will be safer after URI resolves.

Case 4

A 6-week-old boy is brought to the emergency center with a right groin mass first noted when the infant became fussy and vomited.

OBJECTIVE 1

The student should elicit further history from the parents.
  A. Previous inguinal swelling (none).

  B. Birth (infant born at 34 weeks' gestation).
  C. Neonatal problems (required ventilator for hyaline membrane disease).
  D. Neonatal hospitalization (discharged from the neonatal intensive care unit [NICU] 2 weeks ago).
  E. Other (has apnea and is on a monitor at home).

OBJECTIVE 2

The student should perform an appropriate physical examination.
  A. General (small, irritable infant).
  B. Vital signs (tympanic temperature, 37.5°C; weight, 3 kg; pulse, 160/minute; respiratory rate, 50/minute; BP, 75/45 mm Hg).
  C. Chest (lungs clear, heart without murmur).
  D. Abdomen (slightly distended, soft without masses).
  E. Genital examination (firm, slightly tender, walnut-sized mass at the right external ring).

OBJECTIVE 3

The student should diagnose an incarcerated inguinal hernia and describe appropriate initial diagnostic and therapeutic management.
  A. CBC (Hb 9.9 g/dL, Hct 30%, WBC 19,000/mm^3, segs 73%, bands 14%, lymphs 13%, platelets 250,000/mm^3).
  B. Electrolytes (Na, 143 mEq/L; K, 3.9 mEq/L).
  C. Urinalysis (ketones 1+, sp gr 1.021, negative dipstick).
  D. Abdominal x-ray (dilated small bowel with air-fluid levels).
  E. Genital examination (incarcerated right inguinal hernia reduced with sustained gentle pressure toward internal ring).

OBJECTIVE 4

The student should describe appropriate further management.
  A. Hospital admission.
  B. Continuous cardiac and apnea monitoring.
  C. Nothing by mouth (NPO) and nasogastric sump.
  D. Intravenous administration at more than maintenance rate (dextrose 5% [D$_5$] with 1/4 or 1/2 normal saline [NS] at 15–25 mL/hr).
  E. Right inguinal hernia repair and left inguinal exploration under spinal anesthesia the next day.

Achievement Level

OBJECTIVE 1

Minimum Level of Achievement for Passing

The student should:
  A. Obtain history from infant's parents.

B. Elicit history of prematurity.
C. Ask about neonatal hospitalization.

Honors Level of Achievement

The student should:
A. Elicit history of apnea and home monitor.
B. Already be considering the possibility of incarcerated hernia.

OBJECTIVE 2

Minimum Level of Achievement for Passing

The student should:
A. Obtain vital signs and weight.
B. Examine infant for signs of bowel obstruction.
C. Palpate mass and both testes.

Honors Level of Achievement

The student should:
A. Recognize normal vital signs with slight fever.
B. Know that infant hernias frequently present incarcerated.

OBJECTIVE 3

Minimum Level of Achievement for Passing

The student should:
A. Diagnose incarcerated inguinal hernia.
B. Order HPD/CBC and urinalysis (electrolytes and abdominal x-rays optional).
C. Obtain early surgical consultation.

Honors Level of Achievement

The student should:
A. Describe technique for reduction of incarceration.
B. Know that testis may be ischemic.

OBJECTIVE 4

Minimum Level of Achievement for Passing

The student should:
A. Admit infant until hernia is repaired.
B. Keep patient NPO until bowel function is assured.
C. Order appropriate i.v. fluids for rehydration.

Honors Level of Achievement

The student should:
A. Order continuous cardiac and apnea monitoring.
B. Recommend spinal anesthesia to decrease apnea risk.

Case 5

A 9-month-old boy is sent to your office because the public health nurse noted that only one testis was in the scrotum.

OBJECTIVE 1

The student should elicit further history from the mother.
A. Mother (young and single).
B. Son's health (otherwise healthy).
C. Testis at birth (does not know if testis was in the scrotum at birth; his newborn hospital record is in another state).
D. Testis observed (never seen testis in the scrotum during bath time or sleep, or noted any inguinal or scrotal swelling).
E. Immunizations (not up to date).

OBJECTIVE 2

The student should perform an appropriate physical examination:
A. General (well-nourished boy with dirty fingernails).
B. Vital signs (tympanic temperature, 37.1°C; weight, 10 kg; pulse, 130/minute; respiratory rate, 30/minute).
C. Chest (lungs clear, heart without murmur).
D. Abdomen (soft without palpable mass).
E. Genital examination (normal left testis in the scrotum, right testis palpable at the external ring but cannot be brought into scrotum).

OBJECTIVE 3

The student should diagnose an undescended testis and describe appropriate management.
A. Orchiopexy if testis not descended by 1 year of age.
B. Distinguish retractile from undescended testis.
C. Undescended testis has an associated hernia sac — tell mother what to watch for (incarceration).
D. Consider the possibility of child neglect.
E. Inform public health nurse of diagnosis and importance of follow-up.

Achievement Level

OBJECTIVE 1

Minimum Level of Achievement for Passing

The student should:
A. Obtain history from infant's mother.
B. Ask if testis has ever been in the scrotum.
C. Elicit birth and immunization history.

Honors Level of Achievement

The student should:
- A. Ask for newborn records.
- B. Question for associated inguinal hernia.

OBJECTIVE 2

Minimum Level of Achievement for Passing

The student should:
- A. Obtain vital signs and weight.
- B. Perform thorough physical examination.
- C. Palpate both testes.

Honors Level of Achievement

The student should:
- A. Have patient sit with legs crossed for examination.
- B. Notice good nutrition and poor hygiene.

OBJECTIVE 3

Minimum Level of Achievement for Passing

The student should:
- A. Diagnose undescended testis.
- B. Know timing of and reasons for orchiopexy.
- C. Differentiate undescended from retractile testes.

Honors Level of Achievement

The student should:
- A. Educate mother about appearance of associated hernia.
- B. Consider child neglect and arrange close follow-up.

Case 6

A 6-month-old girl is seen in clinic for alternating irritability and lethargy.

OBJECTIVE 1

The student should elicit further history from the parents.
- A. Pain (intermittent for 24 hours; sometimes associated with retching).
- B. Oral intake (poor).
- C. Last void (12 hours ago).
- D. Stool (normal before onset of pain; none since).

OBJECTIVE 2

The student should perform an appropriate physical examination.
- A. General (apathetic infant who suddenly doubles up and screams).
- B. Vital signs (tympanic temperature, 38.2°C; weight, 8 kg; pulse, 175/minute; respiratory rate, 33/minute; BP, 80/55 mm Hg).
- C. Chest (lungs clear, heart sounds normal).
- D. Abdomen (distended, tympanitic, no mass palpable).
- E. Rectum (no mass, bloody mucus).

OBJECTIVE 3

The student should suspect intussusception and order appropriate laboratory and x-ray studies.
- A. CBC (WBC 18,000/mm^3, segs 72%, bands 25%, lymphs 3%, Hct 38%, Hgb 12 g/dL, platelets 184,000/mm^3).
- B. Urinalysis (ketones 2+, sp gr 1.024, negative microscopic).
- C. Electrolytes (Na, 136 mEq/L; K, 4 mEq/L).
- D. Chest x-ray (lung fields clear).
- E. Abdominal x-ray (dilated small bowel, no air in rectum).
- F. Contrast enema (intussusception reduced into cecum).

OBJECTIVE 4

The student should outline preoperative preparations.
- A. Start i.v. of lactated Ringer's at 80–160 mL/hr.
- B. Administer i.v. antibiotics (gentamicin and clindamycin or metronidazole).
- C. Insert nasogastric sump and begin suction.
- D. Obtain informed operative consent from parents: reduction or resection, with appendectomy.

Achievement Level

OBJECTIVE 1

Minimum Level of Achievement for Passing

The student should:
- A. Obtain history from parents.
- B. Elicit duration of pain and associated retching.
- C. Perform gastrointestinal review of symptoms.

Honors Level of Achievement

The student should:
- A. Ask the time and concentration of last void.
- B. Already be considering possibility of intussusception.

OBJECTIVE 2

Minimum Level of Achievement for Passing

The student should:
- A. Obtain visual assessment, vital signs, and weight.
- B. Perform complete abdominal examination, in correct order.
- C. Examine rectum.

Honors Level of Achievement

The student should:
  A. Recognize signs of intestinal obstruction.
  B. Identify dehydration.

OBJECTIVE 3

Minimum Level of Achievement for Passing

The student should:
  A. Suspect intussusception and arrange contrast enema.
  B. Order CBC, urinalysis, electrolytes, and abdominal films.
  C. Initiate i.v. rehydration.

Honors Level of Achievement

The student should:
  A. Identify left shift and dehydration.
  B. Obtain surgical consultation before contrast enema.

OBJECTIVE 4

Minimum Level of Achievement for Passing

The student should:
  A. Start 10–20 mL/kg lactated Ringer's bolus.
  B. Order antibiotics effective against enteric organisms.
  C. Establish continuous nasogastric decompression.

Honors Level of Achievement

The student should:
  A. Realize resection may be necessary.
  B. Know perforation more likely in infants under 6 months of age.

Case 7

A 4-week-old boy is brought to your office after vomiting intermittently for a week, and after every feeding during the past 24 hours.

OBJECTIVE 1

The student should elicit further history from the parents.
  A. Appetite (infant is breast fed and acts hungry all the time).
  B. Vomitus (forceful and never contains bile).
  C. Last void (7 hours ago).
  D. Weight (4.5 kg at 2-week check-up).
  E. Birth weight (4 kg, normal pregnancy and delivery).

OBJECTIVE 2

The student should perform an appropriate physical examination.
  A. General (thin, ravenous infant not satisfied by pacifier).
  B. Vital signs (tympanic temperature, 36.9°C; weight, 4 kg; pulse, 148/minute; respiratory rate, 42/minute; BP, 90/44 mm Hg).
  C. Head, eyes, ears, nose, throat (normal).
  D. Chest (clear lungs, heart sounds normal).
  E. Abdomen (initially, infant crying and epigastrium distended — unable to palpate; after nasogastric sump, sugar on pacifier, and hip flexion — soft, nondistended, normal bowel sounds, palpable olive in upper abdomen).
  F. Rectum (normal, not necessary).

OBJECTIVE 3

The student should suspect pyloric stenosis and order the appropriate laboratory studies.
  A. CBC (WBC 14,200/mm^3, segs 24%, bands 0, lymphs 67%, monos 9%, Hct 35%, Hgb 11.4 g/dL, platelets 346,000/mm^3).
  B. Urinalysis (ketones 2+, sp gr 1.018, negative microscopic).
  C. Electrolytes (Na, 136 mEq/L; K, 4.7 mEq/L; chloride [Cl], 98 mEq/L; CO_2, 22 mEq/L).
  D. Chest x-ray (lung fields clear, unnecessary).
  E. Abdominal x-ray (dilated stomach, unnecessary).
  F. Abdominal ultrasound, if physical examination inadequate (pyloric muscle wall thickness 4.5 mm and pyloric channel length 20 mm — diagnostic for pyloric stenosis).

OBJECTIVE 4

The student should outline preoperative preparations and subsequent care.
  A. Start D$_5$ 1/2 NS and 20 mEq KCl/L at 20–30 mL/hr.
  B. Maintain nasogastric sump on suction.
  C. Pyloromyotomy.
  D. Begin gradually increasing oral intake 12 hours postoperatively.

Achievement Level

OBJECTIVE 1

Minimum Level of Achievement for Passing

The student should:
  A. Obtain history from parents.
  B. Elicit specific information about vomiting.
  C. Acquire birth and immunization history.

Honors Level of Achievement

The student should:
  A. Compare weights and recognize failure to thrive.

B. Include pyloric stenosis and gastroesophageal reflux in the differential diagnosis.

OBJECTIVE 2

Minimum Level of Achievement for Passing

The student should:
A. Make visual assessment, noting hunger.
B. Obtain vital signs and weight.
C. Perform a complete examination, including abdominal palpation.

Honors Level of Achievement

The student should:
A. Empty the infant's stomach, quiet him, and flex his hips.
B. Diagnose pyloric stenosis by palpation of the olive.

OBJECTIVE 3

Minimum Level of Achievement for Passing

The student should:
A. Suspect pyloric stenosis or gastroesophageal reflux.
B. Order CBC, urinalysis, and electrolyte tests.
C. Obtain abdominal ultrasound (unless olive was palpated).

Honors Level of Achievement

The student should:
A. Recognize the brief preoperative preparation required.
B. Understand hypochloremic alkalosis of delayed diagnosis.

OBJECTIVE 4

Minimum Level of Achievement for Passing

The student should:
A. Initiate i.v. of D_5 1/2 NS at greater than maintenance rate.
B. Maintain nasogastric decompression.
C. Expedite early pyloromyotomy.

Honors Level of Achievement

The student should:
A. Understand the distinction between pyloromyotomy and pyloroplasty.
B. Anticipate discharge on second postoperative day.

Case 8

A 6-year-old girl presents with recent onset of a tender neck swelling.

OBJECTIVE 1

The student should elicit further history from the child and her parents.
A. Other symptoms (runny nose and sore throat for several days).
B. Temperature (patient felt warm, but temperature not taken).
C. Previous mass (none noted there).
D. Teeth (not painful).
E. Past medical history (negative).

OBJECTIVE 2

The student should perform an appropriate physical examination.
A. General (uncomfortable child holding neck stiff).
B. Vital signs (tympanic temperature, 38.7°C; weight, 22 kg; pulse, 100/minute; respiratory rate, 24/minute).
C. Head, eyes, ear, nose, throat (poorly circumscribed, nonfluctuant, red, tender swelling right lateral neck; clear nasal discharge; tympanic membranes normal; minimal pharyngeal erythema; tonsils enlarged without exudate; teeth and gums normal).
D. Chest (coarse upper airway noise, heart normal).
E. Abdomen (normal, not essential).

OBJECTIVE 3

The student should diagnose a cervical infection and describe appropriate initial diagnostic and therapeutic management.
A. HPD/CBC (WBC 16,000/mm³, segs 71%, bands 18%, lymphs 11%, Hgb 13.5 g/dL, Hct 40%, platelets 300,000/mm³, not mandatory).
B. Urinalysis (negative dipstick, sp gr 1.011, not essential).
C. Chest x-ray (lung fields clear, not essential).
D. Prescription (Rx — broad-spectrum oral antibiotic).
E. Follow-up (return appointment in 3–5 days).

OBJECTIVE 4

The student should reevaluate the patient at the follow-up visit and describe appropriate further treatment. (The examiner may select: 1. improved or 2. unimproved.)
A. History
   1. Child feels much better and is afebrile.
   2. Neck still swollen and sore; low-grade fever.
B. Physical examination
   1. Happy child with smaller nontender mass right neck.
   2. Unhappy child not moving neck, tympanic temperature 38.2°C, circumscribed tender

swelling right neck, ears-nose-throat [ENT] normal, chest clear.
- C. Appropriate diagnostic studies
  1. None indicated.
  2. Ultrasound if unable to detect fluctuance: abscess.
- D. Therapeutic management
  1. Continue oral antibiotic, schedule return visit to examine for preexisting mass requiring excision.
  2. Incision and drainage with antibiotic coverage, anesthesia, informed consent, and follow-up.

Achievement Level

OBJECTIVE 1

Minimum Level of Achievement for Passing

The student should:
- A. Obtain history from patient and accompanying adults.
- B. Ask about associated symptoms, including fever.
- C. Elicit past medical history.

Honors Level of Achievement

The student should:
- A. Consider infection of preexisting lesion.
- B. Recognize possible dental etiology.

OBJECTIVE 2

Minimum Level of Achievement for Passing

The student should:
- A. Make visual assessment of child, including movement.
- B. Obtain vital signs and weight.
- C. Perform head, eyes, ear, nose, throat, and chest examination.

Honors Level of Achievement

The student should:
- A. Look for signs of preexisting lesion, including sinus tract.
- B. Examine teeth and gums thoroughly.

OBJECTIVE 3

Minimum Level of Achievement for Passing

The student should:
- A. Diagnose cervical cellulitis.
- B. Request laboratory studies (optional).
- C. Prescribe broad-spectrum oral antibiotic.
- D. Schedule early return appointment.

Honors Level of Achievement

The student should:
- A. Include infected nodes, branchial cyst, or lymphangioma in differential diagnosis.

- B. Know that *Staphylococcus aureus* is the most common organism.

OBJECTIVE 4

Minimum Level of Achievement for Passing

The student should:
- A. Elicit interval history
- B. Perform limited physical examination.
- C. Order indicated diagnostic tests.
- D. Obtain appropriate therapy and follow-up.

Honors Level of Achievement

The student should:
- A. 2. Order ultrasound if fluctuance not palpable.
- B. 1 and 2. Continue to look for preexisting lesion.
  2. Select appropriate antibiotic coverage and anesthesia; obtain informed consent.

Case 9

A 3-year-old boy is brought to the emergency center with bleeding per rectum.

OBJECTIVE 1

The student should elicit further history from the parents:
- A. Amount (his mother says it filled the toilet bowl).
- B. Previous bleeding problems (none).
- C. Past medical history and review of systems (negative).
- D. Immunizations (current).
- E. History of trauma (none).

OBJECTIVE 2

The student should perform an appropriate physical examination.
- A. General (pale, wary child, who does not appear in pain; capillary refill normal).
- B. Vital signs (tympanic temperature, 36.7°C; weight, 15 kg; pulse, 125/minute; respiratory rate, 25/minute; BP, 90/60 mm Hg).
- C. Head, eyes, ears, nose, throat (no blood in nose, no loose teeth, no signs of oral trauma).
- D. Chest (heart sounds normal, lungs clear).
- E. Abdomen (cutaneous veins normal, soft and tender, increased bowel sounds, no organomegaly).
- F. Rectum (no hemorrhoids or masses, strongly guaiac-positive, brick-red material).
- G. Nasogastric aspirate (clear, guaiac-negative fluid).

OBJECTIVE 3

The student should diagnose a lower gastrointestinal bleed and describe appropriate diagnostic and therapeutic management.
  A. CBC (WBC 9,500/mm^3, neuts 49%, bands 1%, lymphs 50%, Hct 27%, Hgb 9%, platelets 200,000/mm^3).
  B. Urinalysis (dipstick negative, sp gr 1.016).
  C. Electrolytes (normal, not essential).
  D. Clotting studies (prothrombin time [PT] 11.6/sec, partial thromboplastin time [PTT] 33.8/sec).
  E. Type and cross-match (packed red blood cells [RBCs]).
  F. Meckel's technetium scan (positive).

Achievement Level
OBJECTIVE 1

Minimum Level of Achievement for Passing

The student should:
  A. Obtain history from parents.
  B. Attempt to quantify volume of bleed.
  C. Elicit past medical history and review of symptoms, including bleeding diathesis and liver disease.

Honors Level of Achievement

The student should:
  A. Ask about nosebleed, loose teeth, and oral trauma.
  B. Already be considering possibility of Meckel's diverticulum.

OBJECTIVE 2

Minimum Level of Achievement for Passing

The student should:
  A. Obtain visual assessment, vital signs, and weight.
  B. Perform abdominal and rectal examination.
  C. Check nasogastric aspirate.

Honors Level of Achievement

The student should:
  A. Examine nose and mouth thoroughly.
  B. Include an assessment of cutaneous veins and splenic size in abdominal examination.
  C. Include an assessment for hemorrhoids in rectal examination.

OBJECTIVE 3

Minimum Level of Achievement for Passing

The student should:
  A. Diagnose lower gastrointestinal bleed.
  B. Order CBC, urinalysis, clotting studies, and type and cross-match.
  C. Order Meckel's technetium scan.

Honors Level of Achievement

The student should:
  A. Include Meckel's diverticulum and juvenile polyp in the differential diagnosis.
  B. Know that most bleeding Meckel's diverticula contain ectopic gastric mucosa.

Case 10

A 6-hour-old boy presents drooling and with signs of mild respiratory distress.

OBJECTIVE 1

The student should elicit further history from the parents and the primary care physician.
  A. Prenatal (good care; mild, late hypertension).
  B. Delivery (cesarean section at 41 weeks' gestation).
  C. Evaluation (Apgar scores of 7 and 9; required suctioning).
  D. Feeding (would not latch onto breast).
  E. Urine or stool (none).

OBJECTIVE 2

The student should perform an appropriate physical examination:
  A. General (large infant blowing bubbles).
  B. Vital signs (rectal temperature, 36.5°C; weight, 4.8 kg; pulse, 138/minute; respiratory rate, 60/minute; BP 75/50 mm Hg; pulse oximeter, 95% on room air).
  C. Head, eyes, ears, nose, throat (fontanelles soft, red reflexes present, external ears normal in shape and location, palate intact).
  D. Chest (upper airway noises that clear with suctioning, heart regular without murmur).
  E. Abdomen (soft without masses, bowel sounds normal, three vessels in cord).
  F. Rectum (anus patent and in normal location).
  G. Genitourinary system (testes descended bilaterally, uncircumcised).
  H. Musculoskeletal system (no limb defect).
  I. Nasogastric tube (will not pass into stomach).

OBJECTIVE 3

The student should make the diagnosis of esophageal atresia and order appropriate laboratory and x-ray studies.
  A. CBC (WEB 21,600/mm^3. Hgb 17.5 g/dL, Hct 54%, polys 59%, lymphs 28%, monos 6%, eos 1%, meta 1%, platelets 275,000/mm^3).
  B. Urinalysis (sp gr 1.011, dipstick negative).
  C. Electrolytes (Na 138 mEq/L, K 5.5 mEq/L, Calcium 8 mEq/L).

D. Chest-x-ray (lungs clear, heart of normal shape and size, thymic shadow present, bones normal, air in stomach; tip of nasogastric tube in place just above carina).
E. Abdominal x-ray (air in proximal bowel).

OBJECTIVE 4

The student should diagnose esophageal atresia with distal tracheoesophageal fistula, outline preoperative preparations, and screen for associated VACTERL (vertebral, anorectal, cardiac, tracheal, esophageal, renal, and limb) anomalies.
A. Start i.v. of D_5 1/4 NS at 16–20 mL/hr.
B. Administer i.v. antibiotics.
C. Inform parents: possible VACTERL-associated anomalies; possible tracheomalacia and/or gastroesophageal reflux postoperatively.
D. Perform renal ultrasound.
E. Consult with a cardiologist, as necessary, regarding a murmur or oxygen requirement.

Achievement Level

OBJECTIVE 1

Minimal Level of Achievement of Passing

The student should:
A. Handle the patient emergently.
B. Take history from parents and infant's physician.
C. Ask about birth resuscitation and subsequent intake.

Honors Level of Achievement

The student should:
A. Ask about voiding.
B. Already be considering the possibility of esophageal atresia.

OBJECTIVE 2

Minimal Level of Achievement for Passing

The student should:
A. Include congenital anomaly assessment in the physical examination.
B. Recognize elevated respiratory rate.
C. Try to pass nasogastric tube.

Honors Level of Achievement

The student should already be evaluating for VACTERL-associated anomalies.

OBJECTIVE 3

Minimum Level of Achievement for Passing

The student should:
A. Recognize the probability of esophageal atresia.
B. Order stat chest x-ray.

Honors Level of Achievement

The student should:
A. Recognize all laboratory values as normal for a newborn.
B. Interpret chest x-ray efficiently.

OBJECTIVE 4

Minimum Level of Achievement for Passing

The student should:
A. Diagnose esophageal atresia with tracheoesophageal fistula.
B. Keep patient n.p.o. and start i.v. fluids.
C. Know components of VACTERL association and workup for each.

Honors Level of Achievement

The student should:
A. Elevate the head of the bed to prevent gastroesophageal reflux.
B. Know tracheomalacia is a potential problem.

Case 11

A previously healthy 10-day-old girl presents with bilious vomiting of 12 hours' duration.

OBJECTIVE 1

The student should elicit further history from the parents.
A. Prenatal (negative).
B. Delivery (vaginal at 40 weeks' gestation).
C. Feeding (breast-feeding well until today).
D. Stooling (stooling several times a day until today).
E. Voiding (voiding well until today).

OBJECTIVE 2

The student should perform an appropriate physical examination:
A. General (well-nourished, irritable infant).
B. Vital signs (tympanic temperature, 37.3°C; weight, 4.5 kg; pulse, 170/minute; respiratory rate, 30/minute; BP, 70/45 mm Hg).
C. Head, eyes, ears, nose, throat (PERRL, EOMI, neck supple, fontanelle soft, bilateral red reflex, pharynx clear).
D. Chest (heart regular without murmur, lungs clear without retractions).
E. Abodmen (soft and flat, bowel sounds present, no masses or tenderness).
F. Rectum (patent without masses, stool guaiac negative).

OBJECTIVE 3

The student should treat the patient emergently and order appropriate laboratory and x-ray studies.
- A. Urinalysis (sp gr 1.019, + ketones).
- B. Start i.v. of D5/LF at 35–40 mL/hr.
- C. Abdominal x-ray (stomach and duodenum distended, air throughout small and large bowel).
- D. Insert nasogastric sump and place it to suction.
- E. CBC (WBC 11,400/mm^3, Hct 48%, Hb 15.9 g/dL, polys 55%, bands 2%, lymphs 42%, monos 1%, platelets 252,000/mm^3).
- F. Electrolytes (Na, 137 mEq/L; K, 5.4 mEq/L).
- G. Chest x-ray (normal, not necessary).
- H. Emergent barium enema (all of colon in left abdomen; unable to fill cecum).

OBJECTIVE 4

The student should diagnose malrotation with midgut volvulus and outline urgent preoperative preparations.
- A. Immediate transport to neonatal surgical center.
- B. Administer i.v. antibiotics (gentamicin and clindamycin/metronidazole).
- C. Inform parents (possible bowel resection; possible short bowel syndrome).

Achievement Level

OBJECTIVE 1

Minimum Level of Achievement for Passing

The student should:
- A. Handle the patient emergently.
- B. Ask about intake.
- C. Ask about output of urine and stool.

Honors Level of Achievement

The student should:
- A. Already be considering the possibility of midgut volvulus.
- B. Know that the infant is dehydrated.

OBJECTIVE 2

Minimum Level of Achievement for Passing

The student should:
- A. Recognize an elevated pulse rate.
- B. Perform a thorough examination.

Honors Level of Achievement

The student should know that physical findings are usually normal with early midgut volvulus.

OBJECTIVE 3

Minimum Level of Achievement for Passing

The student should:
- A. Pass nasogastric tube and begin suction.

- B. Start isotonic i.v. hydration with glucose.
- C. Order emergent barium enema.

Honors Level of Achievement

The student should:
- A. Know that plain films often are not helpful with volvulus.
- B. Know that laboratory values are often normal with early midgut volvulus.

OBJECTIVE 4

Minimum Level of Achievement for Passing

The student should:
- A. Diagnose malrotation with midgut volvulus.
- B. Recognize an extreme emergency.
- C. Initiate i.v. antibiotics.

Honors Level of Achievement

The student should:
- A. Obtain early surgical consultation.
- B. Know that prenatal volvulus can result in short bowel syndrome.

Case 12

A 3-hour-old girl presents with persistent respiratory distress.

OBJECTIVE 1

The student should elicit further history from the parents and the primary care physician.
- A. Prenatal (maternal hypertension).
- B. Delivery (vaginal delivery at 37 weeks' gestation).
- C. Evaluation (Apgar scores of 6 and 8).
- D. Respiration (tachypnea since birth; treated with oxygen).

OBJECTIVE 2

The student should perform an appropriate physical examination.
- A. General (tachypneic infant, pink on hood oxygen).
- B. Vital signs (birth weight, 4 kg; rectal temperature, 37°C; pulse, 152/minute; respiratory rate, 80/minute; BP, 63/37 mm Hg; pulse oximeter, 97%).
- C. Head, eyes, ears, nose, throat (moderate caput, fontanelles soft, bilateral red reflex, external ears normal, palate intact, neck supple).
- D. Chest (mild subcostal retractions, breath sounds decreased on left, heart sounds maximal to right of sternum no murmur).

E.   Abdomen (flat, soft without masses, three-vessel cord).
F.   Rectum (anus patent, meconium in diaper).
G.   Musculoskeletal system (extremities and reflexes normal).

OBJECTIVE 3

The student should order a stat chest x-ray.
  X-ray shows air bubbles in left chest, heart shifted to right, right lung clear.

OBJECTIVE 4

The student should diagnose a diaphragmatic hernia and outline urgent preoperative preparations.
  A.   Insert nasogastric sump and place it to suction.
  B.   Start i.v. of D5 / 1/4 NS at 20–35 mL/hr.
  C.   CBC (WBC 23,900 mm Hg, Hgb 20.9 g/dL, Hct 64%, polys 53%, bands 23%, lymphs 10%, monos 14%, platelets 142,000/mm^3).
  D.   Insert arterial line.
  E.   Measure arterial blood gases (pH 7.28, PCO_2 48, PO_2 88, Base deficit minus 7).
  F.   Inform parents (pulmonary hypoplasia and hypertension; ECMO if necessary).

Achievement Level

OBJECTIVE 1

Minimum Level of Achievement for Passing

The student should:
  A.   Handle the patient emergently.
  B.   Take history from parents and infant's physician.
  C.   Recognize infant's oxygen requirement as abnormal.

Honors Level of Achievement

The student should consider the possibility of diaphragmatic hernia.

OBJECTIVE 2

Minimum Level of Achievement for Passing

The student should:
  A.   Recognize respiratory distress.
  B.   Elicit abnormal location of breath and heart sounds.
  C.   Include diaphragmatic hernia and pneumothorax in the differential diagnosis.

Honors Level of Achievement

The student should recognize flat abdomen as sign of diaphragmatic hernia.

OBJECTIVE 3

Minimum Level of Achievement for Passing

The student should order a stat chest x-ray.

Honors Level of Achievement

The student should interpret the chest x-ray efficiently.

OBJECTIVE 4

Minimum Level of Achievement for Passing

The student should:
  A.   Diagnose diaphragmatic hernia.
  B.   Pass nasogastric sump.
  C.   Avoid mask ventilation.

Honors Level of Achievement

The student should:
  A.   Obtain early surgical consultation.
  B.   Understand persistent fetal circulation.

Case 13

A 24-hour-old boy presents with abdominal distention and failure to pass meconium.

OBJECTIVE 1

The student should elicit further history from the parents and the primary care physician.
  A.   Prenatal (uncomplicated term pregnancy).
  B.   Delivery (uneventful vaginal delivery).
  C.   Evaluation (Apgar scores of 8 and 9).
  D.   Feeding (poor breast-feeding).
  E.   Urine (decreased output).
  F.   Other (one episode of bilious vomiting).

OBJECTIVE 2

The student should perform an appropriate physical examination.
  A.   General (irritable, distended infant).
  B.   Vital signs (axillary temperature 36.3°C; weight, 2.8 kg; pulse, 160/minute; respiratory rate, 55/minute; BP, 72/48 mm Hg).
  C.   Head, eyes, ears, nose, throat (fontanelles flat and open, nares patent, palate intact, PERRL).
  D.   Chest (lungs clear to auscultation, decreased diaphragmatic excursion, heart regular with grade I/VI ejection to murmur).
  E.   Abdomen (very distended and tympanitic, nontender, bowel sounds present, unable to assess for masses).
  F.   Rectum (should not be performed before abdominal x-ray because it will dilate aganglionic segment).
  G.   Musculoskeletal system (extremities and back normal).

OBJECTIVE 3

The student should form a differential diagnosis, including Hirschsprung's disease and meconium plug syndrome, and be able to defend each possible diagnosis.

OBJECTIVE 4

The student should order and interpret appropriate laboratory and radiologic studies.
  A. HPD/CBC (Hgb 16 g/dL, Hct 46%, WBC 22,500/mm³, polys 69%, bands 13%, lymphs 16, platelets 310,000/mm³).
  B. Urinalysis (sp gr 1.021, ketones +).
  C. Electrolytes (Na, 136 mEq/L; K, 4.6 mEq/L; Ca, 8.9 mEq/L).
  D. Chest x-ray (no active cardiopulmonary process).
  E. Abdominal x-ray (dilated small and large intestine, no air in rectum).
  F. Barium enema (rectum and sigmoid narrowed with marked proximal distention, meconium plug passed as contrast evacuated; 24-hour film shows contrast retained in descending colon).
  G. Rectal suction biopsy (no ganglia present, hypertrophic nerve fibers).

OBJECTIVE 5

The student should recommend appropriate treatment while awaiting x-ray and pathology results and outline subsequent preoperative preparations.
  A. Start i.v. of D5LR at 20–25 mL/hr until patient hydrated, then decrease to maintenance rate.
  B. Insert nasogastric sump and begin suction.
  C. Inform parents that the infant will require a temporary colostomy.
  D. Administer i.v. antibiotics (gentamicin and clindamycin/metronidazole).

Achievement Level

OBJECTIVE 1

Minimum Level of Achievement for Passing

The student should:
  A. Handle the patient emergently.
  B. Take history from parents and infant's physician.
  C. Elicit input and output, including bile vomit.

Honors Level of Achievement

The student should:
  A. Consider the possibility of Hirschsprung's disease.
  B. Know that the infant is dehydrated.

OBJECTIVE 2

Minimum Level of Achievement for Passing

The student should:
  A. Recognize the elevated respiratory rate.
  B. Suspect distal intestinal obstruction.
  C. Not perform rectal examination before obtaining an abdominal x-ray.

Honors Level of Achievement

The student should:
  A. Realize that abdominal distention is compromising respiration.
  B. Express concern about enterocolitis even without peritonitis.

OBJECTIVE 3

Minimum Level of Achievement for Passing

The student should include Hirschsprung's disease in the differential diagnosis.

Honors Level of Achievement

The student should include Hirschsprung's disease and meconium plug in the differential diagnosis.

OBJECTIVE 4

Minimum Level of Achievement for Passing

The student should:
  A. Obtain abdominal films.
  B. Order a barium enema.
  C. Obtain rectal suction biopsy.
  D. Diagnose Hirschsprung's disease.

Honors Level of Achievement

The student should:
  A. Know the importance of film 24 hours after a barium enema.
  B. Know that Hirschsprung's disease and meconium plug can coexist.

OBJECTIVE 5

Minimum Level of Achievement for Passing

The student should:
  A. Pass nasogastric sump and begin suction.
  B. Start isotonic i.v. hydration with glucose.
  C. Know that the infant will require temporary colostomy.

Honors Level of Achievement

The student should:
  A. Order i.v. antibiotics.
  B. Know the timing of the definitive pull-through.

Case 14

An obstetrician in a small town has just delivered a baby girl with an unexpected abdominal wall defect and calls the tertiary care center for help.

OBJECTIVE 1

The student should elicit appropriate information to make a diagnosis and assess the infant. (The examiner may select: 1. gastroschisis or 2. omphalocele.)
  A. Is there a sac or is intestine exposed?
      1. Exposed
      2. Sac
  B. How does the umbilical cord insert?
      1. Normally
      2. Into sac
  C. How large is the fascial defect?
      1. 3 cm
      2. 6 cm
  D. History (38-week pregnancy, cesarean section for preeclampsia, Apgar scores of 6 and 8).
  E. Physical examination (pink, active infant weighing 3 kg; lungs clear; heart without murmur).
  F. Visible associated defects:
      1. None.
      2. Infant is unusual looking (possible trisomy).

OBJECTIVE 2

The student should recommend urgent treatment and transportation.
  A. Pass nasogastric sump and maintain suction.
  B. Place caudal end of infant in plastic bowel bag up to the axillae (bag can be found in the operating room of most hospitals).
  C. Observe color of bowel and support it through bowel bag if dusky (gastroschisis only).
  D. Start upper extremity i.v. to supply glucose and administer broad-spectrum antibiotics.
  E. Keep infant warm.
  F. Dispatch helicopter with neonatal transport team.

OBJECTIVE 3

The student should describe the conversation with parents and referring physician, particularly the factors affecting prognosis.
  1. If the diagnosis is gastroschisis, parents and physician should be told that intestinal absorption and peristalsis are usually delayed, necessitating prolonged parenteral alimentation. The long-term prognosis is excellent.
  2. If the diagnosis is omphalocele, parents and physician should be told that many infants have multiple concomitant serious anomalies affecting prognosis. Those without cardiac or chromosomal defects usually survive.

Achievement Level
OBJECTIVE 1

Minimum Level of Achievement for Passing

The student should:
  A. Handle the patient emergently.
  B. Distinguish omphalocele from gastroschisis.
  C. Know that omphalocele can be associated with other anomalies.

Honors Level of Achievement

The student should know that trisomy is associated with omphalocele.

OBJECTIVE 2

Minimum Level of Achievement for Passing

The student should:
  A. Pass the nasogastric sump and begin suction.
  B. Place infant's legs and trunk in plastic bowel bag.
  C. Initiate upper extremity i.v. line and antibiotics.
  D. Provide emergent skilled transportation.

Honors Level of Achievement

The student should:
  A. Observe the color of the gastroschisis bowel.
  B. Keep the infant warm.

OBJECTIVE 3

Minimum Level of Achievement for Passing

The student should know the short- and long-term prognosis of each defect.

Honors Level of Achievement

The student should obtain early surgical consultation.

Case 15

A 7-year-old boy was struck by a van while riding his bicycle not far from the hospital. He was not wearing a helmet. At the scene, he was unresponsive, breathing, and acyanotic. There was bleeding from a large scalp laceration and an open left femur fracture. Paramedics applied a head dressing, traction splint, cervical collar, spine board, and oxygen mask. He arrives in the emergency center within 15 minutes of the accident with a pulse of 150/minute, BP of 80 mm Hg, and respiratory rate of 30/minute.

OBJECTIVE 1

The student should perform a primary survey and immediately treat life-threatening conditions.
A. Airway maintenance with cervical spine control (trachea midline, noisy breathing that clears with suction).
B. Breathing and ventilation (breath sounds equal, rapid and shallow; pulse oximeter 100% on oxygen by face mask).
C. Circulation with hemorrhage control (pulse rapid, capillary refill 6 seconds; draw blood for type and cross-match, HPD/CBC, amylase, PT, and PTT while establishing two large-caliber i.v. lines; estimate weight at 22–24 kg and administer immediate 450 mL [20 mL/kg] bolus of *warm* lactated Ringer's).
D. Disability (neurologic status — responsive only to painful stimuli; PERRL).
E. Exposure (completely undress the patient; head dressing starting to soak through so apply direct pressure; left leg in traction; no other external signs of trauma).

OBJECTIVE 2

The student should describe appropriate, immediate diagnostic evaluation and treatment.
A. Electrocardiographic monitoring (sinus tachycardia).
B. Order lateral cervical spine film.
C. Assess for cribriform fracture; pass nasogastric sump and begin suction.
D. Rectal and genital examination (do *not* place Foley catheter before evaluating for urethral trauma).
E. Keep patient warm, covered when possible.

OBJECTIVE 3

The student should perform a secondary survey while continuing appropriate treatment.
A. Vital signs (BP, 90/70 mm/Hg; pulse, 125/minute; respiration, 25/minute; tympanic temperature, 36.5°C; give second bolus of 450 mL lactated Ringer's).
B. Head, eyes, ears, nose, throat (bleeding from scalp laceration controlled, pupils equal and reactive, tympanic membranes and oropharynx clear).
C. Chest (breath sounds remain equal and shallow, heart regular without murmur).
D. Abdomen (nondistended, bowel sounds decreased; rectal and genital examination normal; insert Foley catheter).
E. Extremities and spine (open left femur fracture with bleeding controlled, peripheral pulses present).
F. Neurologic (painful stimulus elicits eye opening, incomprehensible sounds, and appropriate withdrawal in all four extremities — Glasgow coma scale score of 9; PERRL).

OBJECTIVE 4

The student should order, justify, and interpret appropriate laboratory and radiologic studies.
A. Lateral cervical x-ray through 0-7 (no fracture; intubate patient and begin hyperventilation).
B. Chest x-ray (endotracheal tube in good position; lung fields clear).
C. Left femur (displaced fracture).
D. Urinalysis (dipstick negative).
E. HPD/CBC (WBC 15,500/mm^3, Hgb 10.5 g/dL, Hct 32%, platelets 225,000/mm^3).
F. Amylase (67 IU/L).
G. Head CT — continue monitoring (mild diffuse swelling without skull fracture or focal injury).

Achievement Level

OBJECTIVE 1

Minimum Level of Achievement for Passing

The student should rapidly:
A. Clear airway and administer oxygen.
B. Start large-caliber i.v. lines and draw blood for appropriate laboratory studies.
C. Recognize hemorrhagic shock, control external bleeding with direct pressure, and administer isotonic fluid bolus.

Honors Level of Achievement

The student should:
A. Continuously monitor oxygenation.
B. Use warm i.v. fluids.

OBJECTIVE 2

Minimum Level of Achievement for Passing

The student should:
A. Evaluate the cervical spine.
B. Pass nasogastric tube.
C. Perform genital and rectal examination before passing Foley catheter.

Honors Level of Achievement

The student should:
A. Consider the possibility of cribriform fracture.
B. Keep the patient warm.

OBJECTIVE 3

Minimum Level of Achievement for Passing

The student should:
  A. Perform a complete physical examination.
  B. Recognize persistent hypovolemia and repeat fluid bolus.
  C. Perform a genital and rectal examination before inserting a Foley catheter.

Honors Level of Achievement

The student should know the Glasgow coma scale.

OBJECTIVE 4

Minimum Level of Achievement for Passing

The student should:
  A. Diagnose closed-head injury and femur fracture.
  B. Intubate and hyperventilate.
  C. Order lateral cervical spine film, urinalysis, amylase, and HPD/CBC.

Honors Level of Achievement

The student should continuously monitor ECG and ventilation.

Case 16

A 2-year-old girl is brought to the emergency center because she has refused to walk for 2 days.

OBJECTIVE 1

The student should obtain appropriate additional history from the mother and mother's boyfriend, while closely observing their demeanor.
  A. History of injury (none).
  B. Primary care physician (none).
  C. Immunizations (not up to date).
  D. Child care (the child and her older brother are cared for by the boyfriend while the mother works a night shift).
  E. Mother's behavior (appears exhausted).
  F. Child's behavior (clings to her mother).
  G. Boyfriend's behavior (when he returns from parking the car he takes her brother on his lap, but seems distant).

OBJECTIVE 2

The student should perform an appropriate physical examination.
  A. General (the child is wearing only a T-shirt and diaper in cold weather; her fingernails are broken and dirty; there are bruises on her back and buttocks).

  B. Vital signs (tympanic temperature, 36.5°C; weight, 12 kg; pulse, 120/minute; respiratory rate, 25/minute; BP 90/65 mm Hg).
  C. Chest (no cutaneous injury, lungs clear, heart regular without murmur).
  D. Abdomen (no cutaneous injury, normal bowel sounds, no masses or tenderness).
  E. Perineal (no bruising or discharge).
  F. Extremities (tender warm right calf, left leg and both arms without injury).

OBJECTIVE 3

The student should order and interpret appropriate laboratory and radiologic studies.
  A. CBC (Hgb 11, Hct 33, WBC 13,000, platelets 225,000/mm^3).
  B. Urinalysis (sp gr 10.15, dipstick negative).
  C. Electrolytes (not indicated).
  D. Right calf x-ray (midshaft tibial fracture).
  F. Skeletal survey (healing rib fractures)

OBJECTIVE 4

The student should recommend appropriate treatment.
  A. Hospitalization.
  B. Long leg cast.
  C. "Hot line" call to report suspected child abuse.

Achievement Level

OBJECTIVE 1

Minimum Level of Achievement for Passing

The student should:
  A. Elicit appropriate history.
  B. Observe behavior of adult caretakers.
  C. Suspect child abuse as indicated by delay in seeking medical care, delayed immunizations, no history of injury, boyfriend preoccupied.

Honors Level of Achievement

The student should:
  A. Know that age of majority of abused children is 1 month to 3 years old.
  B. Know that stepparent or cohabitant is common abuser.

OBJECTIVE 2

Minimum Level of Achievement for Passing

The student should:
  A. Note the child's poor hygiene and inappropriate clothes.
  B. Note buttock bruising.
  C. Suspect child abuse.

Honors Level of Achievement

The student should:
- A. Know that an abused child may be sad, withdrawn, or frightened.
- B. Know that poor hygiene, inappropriate clothes, failure to thrive, and developmental delay are signs suspicious for abuse.

OBJECTIVE 3

Minimum Level of Achievement for Passing

The student should:
- A. Order right calf films.
- B. Order skeletal survey.
- C. Suspect repeated child abuse: multiple injuries in various stages of healing.

Honors Level of Achievement

The student should know that:
- A. A midshaft fracture in a toddler is common with abuse.
- B. Lesions of different ages are characteristic of abuse.

OBJECTIVE 4

Minimum Level of Achievement for Passing

The student should:
- A. Identify a very high probability of child abuse.
- B. Admit the patient.
- C. Make a "hot line" call to report suspected abuse.

Honors Level of Achievement

The student should know that:
- A. Reporting suspected child abuse is mandatory.
- B. Repeated abuse is common without intervention.

Case 17

A 9-year-old boy is brought to the emergency center by ambulance 1 hour after a motor vehicle accident. He was an unrestrained passenger and was ejected. Paramedics immobilized him on a back board and started an i.v. line. He is alert and his vital signs have been stable.

OBJECTIVE 1

The student should perform a primary survey:
- A. Airway maintenance with cervical spine control (trachea midline, breathing easily).
- B. Breathing and ventilation (good bilateral breath sounds, pulse oximeter 95% on room air).
- C. Circulation with hemorrhage control (palpable pulses, capillary refill 4 seconds).
- D. Disability (neurologic status — alert and complaining of left abdominal and flank pain).
- E. Exposure (completely undress the patient — abrasion of left costal margin and flank).

OBJECTIVE 2

The student should describe appropriate immediate diagnostic evaluation and treatment:
- A. Start second i.v. line, draw blood for laboratory analysis (CBC, amylase, type and cross-match, estimate patient's weight at 26–30 kg, and run lactated Ringer's at 300 mL/hr).
- B. ECG monitoring.
- C. Pass nasogastric sump (patient vomits; roll and suction, controlling cervical spine).
- D. After genital and rectal examination, place Foley catheter; dipstick urine (moderate RBCs).
- E. Keep patient warm, covered when possible.

OBJECTIVE 3

The student should perform a secondary survey:
- A. Vital signs (BP, 100/60 mm Hg; pulse, 110/minute; respiration, 24/minute; tympanic temperature, 36.4°C).
- B. Head, eyes, ears, nose, throat (pupils equal and reactive, extraocular movements intact, tympanic membranes and oropharynx clear, neck nontender).
- C. Chest (tenderness and abrasion over left lower ribs, decreased breath sounds at left base, heart regular without murmur).
- D. Abdomen (nondistended, left upper quadrant tenderness, bowel sounds decreased, rectal examination normal).
- E. Extremities and spine (no deformity or tenderness, peripheral pulses present, no neurologic deficit).
- F. Neurologic (oriented, moves all extremities to command, cranial nerves intact, Glasgow coma scale score of 15).

OBJECTIVE 4

The student should order, justify, and interpret appropriate laboratory and radiologic studies:
- A. Chest x-ray (no rib fractures, slight haziness of left diaphragm).
- B. Urinalysis (250 RBC, sp gr 1.020).
- C. Amylase (100 IU/L).
- D. CBC (WBC 15,200/mm^3, Hgb 12.6 g/dL, Hct 35%, platelets 350,000/mm^3).
- E. Abdominal CT (give metoclopramide, continue monitoring; splenic fracture, contusion upper pole left kidney).

Achievement Level

OBJECTIVE 1

Minimum Level of Achievement for Passing

The student should:
A. Evaluate the airway with cervical spine immobilization.
B. Recognize hypovolemia.
C. Recognize possible abdominal injury.

Honors Level of Achievement

The student should:
A. Obtain early surgical involvement.
B. Measure peripheral oxygenation.

OBJECTIVE 2

Minimum Level of Achievement for Passing

The student should:
A. Initiate vigorous appropriate fluid resuscitation.
B. Log-roll the patient when he vomits.
C. Place Foley catheter and test urine with dipstick.

Honors Level of Achievement

The student should:
A. Draw laboratory tests while starting i.v. line.
B. Keep patient covered when procedures are not being done.
C. Use warm Ringer's lactate.

OBJECTIVE 3

Minimum Level of Achievement for Passing

The student should:
A. Perform complete physical examination.
B. Recognize vital signs as normal for child this age.
C. Perform genital and rectal examination before inserting Foley catheter.

Honors Level of Achievement

The student should recognize possible splenic injury.

OBJECTIVE 4

Minimum Level of Achievement for Passing

The student should:
A. Discuss requirements for nonoperative management.
B. Transport patient to tertiary pediatric trauma center.

Honors Level of Achievement

The student should:
A. Remember to give metoclopramide.

B. Recognize pleural fluid secondary to pulmonary or splenic injury.

Case 18

A 3-year-old boy is brought to clinic because his grandmother thinks his abdomen is becoming too large.

OBJECTIVE 1

The student should elicit further history from the parents and grandmother.
A. Behavior (less energy than usual the past week).
B. Appetite (recent decrease).
C. Weight loss or fever (none known).
D. Other symptoms (no excess catecholamines, no lower extremity weakness, no incontinence).
E. Family observations (grandmother had been on vacation and had not seen him for several weeks before her observation).
F. Delivery and postnatal history (cesarean section for breech presentation; jaundice requiring phototherapy).
G. Respiration (recurrent bronchitis; hospitalized at 15 months for pneumonia).

OBJECTIVE 2

The student should perform an appropriate physical examination.
A. General (anxious boy with distended abdomen, no subcutaneous nodules).
B. Vital signs (weight, 16 kg; tympanic temperature, 36.8°C; BP, 120/70 mm Hg; pulse, 120/minute; respiratory rate, 25/minute).
C. Head, eyes, ears, nose, throat (extraocular movements intact, pupils equally round and reactive, bilateral red reflexes, no proptosis or periorbital ecchymosis, tympanic membranes normal).
D. Chest (breath sounds clear and equal, heart regular without murmur).
E. Abdomen (protuberant, normoactive bowel sounds; nontender, large irregular firm mass on left side inseparable from left kidney or liver).
F. Rectum (normal, no mass palpable).
G. Genital examination (bilateral descended testes without hernia).
H. Nodes (shoddy cervical and inguinal nodes, no axillary nodes).
I. Central nervous system (cranial nerves II-XII intact, normal motor and sensory exam, deep tendon reflexes 2/4).

OBJECTIVE 3

The student should form a differential diagnosis (in order of probability) and be able to defend each possible diagnosis.
  A. Neuroblastoma.
  B. Wilms'' tumor.
  C. Malignant hepatic tumor.

OBJECTIVE 4

The student should order and interpret appropriate laboratory and x-ray studies.
  A. CBC(WBC 15,500/mm^3, Hgb 13.9 g/dL, Hct 40%, platelets 242,000/mm^3, differential normal).
  B. Urinalysis (sp gr 1.018, + ketones, rest of dipstick negative).
  C. SMAC (BUN, 10 mg/dL; creatinine, 0.7 mg/dL; albumin, 3.1 g/dL; inorganic phosphorus, 5.8 mg/dL; alkaline phosphatase, 300 IU/L).
  D. Bone marrow (normal).
  E. Chest x-ray (cardiomediastinal silhouette, lungs and bony thorax are unremarkable).
  F. Abdominal ultrasound (large mass lesion continuous with upper pole of left kidney).
  G. Abdominal CT (large left suprarenal mass lesion with calcifications, poor visualization of the inferior vena cava, no evidence of other mass or lymphadenopathy).
  H. Bone scan (no skeletal metastases).

OBJECTIVE 5

The student should refer the patient to a pediatric oncologist (or surgeon associated with a pediatric oncology study group) for surgery and chemotherapy by protocol.

Achievement Level

OBJECTIVE 1

Minimum Level of Achievement for Passing

The student should:
  A. Elicit decreased energy level.
  B. Elicit depressed appetite.
  C. Ask about weight loss and fever.

Honors Level of Achievement

The student:
  A. Is already considering neuroblastoma and Wilms' tumor.
  B. Asks about symptoms of catecholamine excess, lower extremity weakness, and incontinence.

OBJECTIVE 2

Minimum Level of Achievement for Passing

The student should:
  A. Perform a thorough examination, including nodes and rectum.
  B. Recognize vital signs as normal.

Honors Level of Achievement

The student should:
  A. Recognize irregularity as more consistent with neuroblastoma.
  B. Look for subcutaneous nodules, proptosis, periorbital ecchymosis, and lower extremity weakness.

OBJECTIVE 3

Minimum Level of Achievement for Passing

The student should be able to list the top three possibilities.

Honors Level of Achievement

The student should be able to rank the top three possibilities.

OBJECTIVE 4

Minimum Level of Achievement for Passing

The student should:
  A. Obtain bone marrow.
  B. Order abdominal ultrasound.
  C. Order abdominal CT when ultrasound results available.

Honors Level of Achievement

The student should:
  A. Know calcifications are common in neuroblastoma.
  B. Order chest x-ray and bone scan.
  C. Know inorganic phosphorus and alkaline phosphatase are normal for age.

OBJECTIVE 5

Minimum Level of Achievement for Passing

The student should:
  A. Know about national randomized tumor protocols.
  B. Know that child is best treated by pediatric oncologic specialists familiar with staging requirements.

Honors Level of Achievement

The student should know about late complications of therapy and need for long-term follow-up.

3

Ophthalmology: Diseases of the Eye

Case 1

You are an ophthalmologist, and a young woman presents with a history of pain and foreign body sensation in her left eye that has occurred about six times in the last few months, especially on awakening. These symptoms tend to resolve over the first 6 hours after she notes her symptoms. She has no complaints with the right eye.

OBJECTIVE 1

The student should discuss further historical information to be obtained.
 A. History of eye trauma (yes; scratch from baby's fingernail resulting in a corneal abrasion left eye [OS] 1 year ago).
 B. Contact lens use (no).
 C. Similar family history (no).
 D. General medical history, specifically rheumatoid disease, Sjögren's with dry eye (no).

OBJECTIVE 2

The student should outline specific findings being sought on examination.
 A. Foreign body (no).
 B. Corneal abrasion or erosion (yes, inferior to the visual axis).
 C. Corneal dystrophies in either eye (yes, fingerprint lines in the corneal epithelium in both eyes, worse in the left).
 D. Dry eye syndrome, corneal changes (no).
 E. Eyelid abnormalities resulting in corneal exposure with closed lids (no).

OBJECTIVE 3

A diagnosis is made of recurrent corneal erosion of the left eye, associated with prior trauma as well as map-dot-fingerprint corneal dystrophy. The examination is otherwise normal. The left eye is patched with an antibiotic ointment and heals over the next 2 days. The patient now requests treatment so that the corneal erosion does not recur. The student should outline a treatment plan, as well as the next step should the current treatment fail, and explain the rationale for each.
 A. Topical lubricants (low risk, easy, and often effective).
 B. Topical hypertonic saline medications (low risk, easy, and often effective).
 C. Patching at night (low risk, easy, and often effective).
 D. Bandage contact lens (small risk, easy, and often effective).
 E. Debridement of corneal epithelium at the site of the erosion (more effective than above treatments for persistent erosions; small risk but increased patient discomfort for a couple of days).
 F. Anterior stromal puncture to the site of the erosion (increased effectiveness for persistent erosions, but faint scars will be produced, patient will have initial discomfort, and treatment carries small risk of perforation, infection, visual disturbances).

Achievement Level

OBJECTIVE 1

Minimum Level of Achievement for Passing

The student should:
 A. Obtain other important historical information, at least regarding a history of trauma.
 B. Rule out a history of foreign body or activities risky for trauma (such as grinding metal).

Honors Level of Achievement

The student should:
 A. Discuss the association of some inherited corneal dystrophies with recurrent erosions.
 B. Rule out associated systemic conditions with dry eye syndrome.

OBJECTIVE 2

Minimum Level of Achievement for Passing

The student should:
- A. Rule out a foreign body on examination.
- B. Examine specifically for a corneal abrasion/ erosion.

Honors Level of Achievement

The student should:
- A. Examine for corneal dystrophies in either eye (specifically map-dot-fingerprint and lattice dystrophies).
- B. Rule out eyelid abnormalities and dry eye syndrome changes on examination.

OBJECTIVE 3

Minimum Level of Achievement for Passing

The student should be able to provide a stepwise treatment, explain the rationale, and include at least three specific treatments.

Honors Level of Achievement

The student should be able to explain the procedure of anterior stromal puncture and its risks.

Case 2

A 75-year-old female presents to your ophthalmologic office in New York for a second opinion regarding her "need" for a corneal transplant in her right eye, as told to her by another local ophthalmologist (a retinal specialist who states that the patient's retinas and optic nerves are normal). The patient feels her vision has become worse in her right eye over the last year, with vision in her left eye worsening as well.

OBJECTIVE 1

The student should outline an initial evaluation of the patient, history, and anterior segment eye examination, eliciting pertinent information.
- A. History of previous eye surgery (yes; cataract surgery right eye only while vacationing in Florida last year).
- B. History of trauma (no).
- C. Family history of corneal disease/surgery (yes, her brother had both corneas transplanted when he was 65 years old).
- D. Best corrected visual acuity (20/100 right eye [OD] and 20/50 OS).
- E. Intraocular pressures (16 mm Hg in each eye, normal up to 21 mm Hg).
- F. Anterior segment examined for:
  1. Corneal opacities or edema (edema; OD greater than OS).
  2. Lens implants, cataracts (yes; a well-placed, stable posterior chamber lens implant OD with a mild, visually insignificant cataract OS).
  3. Evidence of corneal dystrophies (yes, corneal guttae in both eyes).

OBJECTIVE 2

The student should discuss a differential diagnosis, any further testing, and a treatment plan.
- A. Differential diagnosis should include Fuch's dystrophy, pseudophakic bullous keratopathy, Fuch's dystrophy worsened by cataract surgery.
- B. Specular microscopy (300 cells/mm^2 OD and 600 cells/mm^2 OS).
- C. Corneal pachymetry (central corneal thickness 0.72 mm OD and 0.65 mm OS).
- D. Trial of hypertonic saline medications in an attempt to dehydrate the patient's corneas (likely to fail OD).
- E. Gentle forced air from a hair dryer blown over the patient's corneas to decrease the edema (likely to fail OD).
- F. Corneal transplantation OD (option of corneal transplantation OS in the future with possible cataract surgery).

OBJECTIVE 3

The student should outline a surgical plan for corneal transplantation OD with postoperative care regimen.
- A. Penetrating (not lamellar) keratoplasty.
- B. Oversized graft by about 1/2 mm.
- C. Suture technique with rationale.
- D. Leave lens implant in place (if indeed found to be stable at the time of surgery).
- E. Long-term postoperative topical steroids (with topical antibiotic for short term).

Additional Questions

1. What important findings in this patient would make her risk of corneal transplant rejection relatively low? (Lack of preoperative inflammation, lack of peripheral corneal vascularization, a relatively favorable diagnosis, older age, normal intraocular pressure, normal ocular adnexa.)

2. What warning signs or symptoms of rejection would you give to your patient? (Pain, redness, conjunctival injection, decreased vision, or no symptoms — i.e., needs regular follow-up.)

3. What are the complications of corneal transplantation? (Infectious keratitis, endophthalmitis, glaucoma, expulsive hemorrhage, wound leaks, retinal detachment, corneal graft rejection, persistent epithelial defects.)

4. What are some other indications for corneal transplantation aside from pseudophakic bullous keratopathy or Fuch's corneal dystrophy? (Corneal

scarring, keratoconus, aphakic bullous keratopathy, virus infections, medically unresponsive infectious keratitis, corneal dystrophies, failed corneal transplants.)

Achievement Level

OBJECTIVE 1

Minimum Level of Achievement for Passing

The student should:
  A. Elicit an accurate history, pointing out important past surgery and lack of eye trauma.
  B. Look specifically for corneal edema or scarring in both eyes.
  C. Note the location and stability of the patient's lens implant.

Honors Level of Achievement

The student should inquire about and note the significance of the positive family history.

OBJECTIVE 2

Minimum Level of Achievement for Passing

The student should:
  A. Include pseudophakic bullous keratopathy in the differential diagnosis.
  B. Include the use of topical hypertonic saline medications and penetrating corneal transplant in the treatment regimen.

Honors Level of Achievement

The student should:
  A. Include specular microscopy and/or corneal pachymetry in further testing.
  B. Include forced air from a hair dryer as a treatment option.

OBJECTIVE 3

Minimum Level of Achievement for Passing

The student should:
  A. Understand the rationale for a full-thickness (penetrating) keratoplasty.
  B. Provide one suturing technique with one of its advantages.
  C. Propose using long-term topical steroids.

Honors Level of Achievement

The student should:
  A. Know to oversize the corneal graft by 1/2 mm and understand that oversizing decreases the risk of postoperative glaucoma.
  B. Choose to leave the current posterior chamber lens implant in place and explain the rationale for doing so.

Additional Questions

Minimum Level of Achievement for Passing

The student should:
  A. Provide at least one reason for a relatively low risk of corneal rejection in this patient.
  B. Provide at least three symptoms of corneal rejection.
  C. Provide two other indications for corneal transplantation.

Honors Level of Achievement

The student should:
  A. Provide at least three reasons for the relatively low risk of corneal rejection in this patient.
  B. Provide at least three other indications for corneal transplantation aside from pseudophakic bullous keratopathy or Fuch's corneal dystrophy.
  C. Provide at least three complications of corneal transplantation (aside from rejection).

Case 3

A young man presents to your ophthalmologic office with a complaint of mildly blurred vision OD. He also notes a long history of small "growths" on the nasal corneas in both eyes for years; he thinks the one OD has grown "slightly." The eye examination is normal except for best corrected vision of 20/25 in each eye and small, noninflamed pterygia 1 and 1/2 mm onto each nasal cornea.

OBJECTIVE 1

The student should obtain further testing to assess the visual effect of the pterygia and further history to help determine therapy.
  A. Patient's level of sun/ultraviolet light exposure (originally from Puerto Rico; currently works outside as a fisherman).
  B. Level of visual disability (having difficulty working because of visual distortion OD).
  C. Keratometry readings (irregular astigmatism, both eyes).
  D. Photokeratoscope evaluation (irregular astigmatism, both eyes; worse OD).

OBJECTIVE 2

The student should outline a treatment plan with accompanying rationale.
  A. Observation (mild current visual disability with relatively high risk of recurrence).
  B. Excision of pterygium OD only (less surgery for first pterygium).

C. Excision of pterygium with conjunctival graft OD (decreased rate of recurrence).
D. Sunglasses (decrease ultraviolet light exposure).

OBJECTIVE 3

The student should propose a different treatment plan if this situation occurs in a patient with a third recurrent pterygium.
A. Observation (same rationale as above).
B. Excision of pterygium with conjunctival graft (decreased rate of recurrence).
C. Excision of pterygium with postoperative treatment using antimetabolite agents (decreased rate of recurrence).
D. Excision of pterygium with use of local postoperative ß-irradiation (decreased rate of recurrence but increased long-term risk of scleral necrosis).

Additional Questions

1. What are some antimetabolite agents that have been used to decrease the rate of pterygium recurrence after excision? (Thiotepa, mitomycin.)
2. What are some complications of pterygium surgery? (Recurrence, conjunctival cicatrization, cicatrization of tissues surrounding extraocular muscles resulting in double vision, corneal scarring, astigmatism.)
3. What are some medical treatments for occasionally inflamed pterygia? (Topical lubricants, vasoconstrictors, and steroids.)

Achievement Level

OBJECTIVE 1

Minimum Level of Achievement for Passing

The student should:
A. Obtain information regarding this patient's ultraviolet light exposure history.
B. Obtain and evaluate information regarding this patient's visual complaint/disability.
C. Obtain an objective measurement of this patient's corneal astigmatism in one manner (keratometer, Placido's disk, or photokeratoscope).

Honors Level of Achievement

The student should obtain objective measurements of the patient's corneal astigmatism in more than one way (keratometer, Placido's disk, or photokeratoscope).

OBJECTIVE 2

Minimum Level of Achievement for Passing

The student should provide at least two treatment options with rationale.

Honors Level of Achievement

The student should provide at least four treatment options with rationale.

OBJECTIVE 3

Minimum Level of Achievement for Passing

The student should provide at least two treatment options with rationale.

Honors Level of Achievement

The student should provide at least four treatment options with rationale.

Additional Questions

Minimum Level of Achievement for Passing

The student should be able to name at least two complications of pterygium excision, excluding infection.

Honors Level of Achievement

The student should be able to name at least:
A. One antimetabolite agent used to prevent recurrence of pterygium.
B. Three complications of pterygium excision, excluding infection.
C. Two nonsurgical treatments for inflamed pterygia.

Case 4

A 64-year-old male presents to your office for evaluation of painless, slowly progressive visual loss.

OBJECTIVE 1

The student should elicit the pertinent history.
A. Trauma (none).
B. Steroid use (none).
C. Diabetes (none).
D. Any other medical causes of visual loss, e.g., multiple sclerosis (none).

OBJECTIVE 2

The student should question the patient concerning the effect of visual loss on the patient's life.
A. Does the patient drive? (Yes.)
B. Can he still drive safely? (No.)
C. Is night vision affected? (Yes.)
D. Can the patient read? (Yes.)
E. What can the patient not do because of poor vision? (Glare causes problems, driving is difficult, night vision is poor.)

OBJECTIVE 3

The student should outline the ophthalmic examination necessary to show that the visual loss is due to cataract formation.
  A. Cornea (normal).
  B. Diabetic retinopathy (fundus examination, normal).
  C. Macular degeneration (fundus examination, normal).
  D. Optic nerve (fundus examination, normal visual field).

OBJECTIVE 4

The student should outline the surgical plan.
  A. Explain the cataract.
  B. Explain surgical procedure.
  C. Explain potential complications.

Achievement Level

Minimum Level of Achievement for Passing

The student should:
  A. Form a reasonable conclusion about visual loss.
  B. Realize the effect of cataracts on the patient's life.
  C. Show that cataract is the main cause of visual loss.
  D. Be able to explain the visual loss to the patient.
  E. Formulate a surgical plan.
  F. Be able to explain the main potential complications.

Honors Level of Achievement

The student should:
  A. Understand the differences between phacoemulsification and extracapsular manual extraction.
  B. Understand the optics involved in cataracts, e.g., a nuclear cataract causes myopia and a "browning effect" while a posterior subcapsular cataract causes glare.

Case 5

A patient who had cataract surgery 28 hours ago presents at the office complaining of a painful eye.

OBJECTIVE 1

The student should be able to outline signs and symptoms associated with endophthalmitis.
  A. Pain (severe, deep ache).
  B. Discharge (profuse).
  C. Color (intense redness).

OBJECTIVE 2

The student should examine for:
  A. Hypopyon (white cells in the anterior chamber).
  B. Vision (decreased).

OBJECTIVE 3

The student should be able to define an appropriate treatment plan that includes:
  A. Tap and culture.
  B. Appropriate antibiotics.

Achievement Level

Minimum Level of Achievement for Passing

The student should:
  A. Be aware that intense pain may signal an infection.
  B. Know the signs of endophthalmitis.

Honors Level of Achievement

The student should:
  A. Know the appropriate antibiotics for each bacteria.
  B. Be able to explain the technique of anterior chamber and vitreous taps.

Case 6

A female patient comes to your office with a red eye. She complains of pain, halos around lights, and nausea.

OBJECTIVE 1

The student should outline the examination and know the differential diagnosis of a red eye.
  A. Vision (red eye, 20/100; other eye 20/20).
  B. Cornea (cloudy).
  C. Pupil (mid-dilated and nonreactive).

OBJECTIVE 2

The student should understand the tests to prove the patient is experiencing a narrow angle glaucoma.
  A. Intraocular pressure (44).
  B. Gonioscopy examination (shows angle to be closed — proof of narrow angle attack).

OBJECTIVE 3

The student should be able to outline treatment:
  A. Drop the intraocular pressure medically (give a drop of Timoptic to reduce aqueous inflow, 500 mg of diazine acetazolamide to reduce aqueous, oral glycerin to remove fluid from the eye osmotically, and a drop of pilocarpine to pull iris away from the cornea).

B. Do a laser iridotomy with either a yittrium aluminum garnert (YAG) laser or an argon laser.

Achievement Level

Minimum Level of Achievement for Passing

The student should:
A. Formulate a reasonable differential diagnosis.
B. Understand the pathophysiology of narrow angle glaucoma.
C. Understand that an iridotomy is indicated.

Honors Level of Achievement

The student should:
A. Understand the use of medications to break a narrow angle attack.
B. Realize that gonioscopy after laser surgery is needed to prove the attack is broken.

Case 7

A 69-year-old male patient that you have been following for glaucoma returns for a visit. His pressure on medication is 26 mm Hg. A visual field examination is done and shows deterioration.

OBJECTIVE 1

The student should understand that even though visual damage from glaucoma usually takes a long period of time (months to years); the pressure of 26 mm Hg is above normal range (22 mm Hg) and must be lowered to a "safe" level.

OBJECTIVE 2

The student should formulate a management plan.
A. If the patient is on a ß-blocker, the student may consider adding an adrenergic drug such as epinephrine or a prodrug (Propine), or a miotic such as pilocarpine. If the patient is already on pilocarpine, the percentage can be increased up to 4%. A systemic carbonic anhydrase inhibitor may also be effective.
B. If the patient is on maximally tolerated medications, the student should consider laser trabeculoplasty.
C. The student should also consider surgical trabeculotomy.

OBJECTIVE 3

The student should be able to describe the appropriate surgical procedures.
A. Laser trabeculoplasty.
B. Trabeculectomy.

Achievement Level

Minimum Level of Achievement for Passing

The student understands the complex relationship between pressure and optic nerve damage.

Honors Level of Achievement

The student understands the complications of trabeculectomy.

Case 8

A 6-month-old girl is brought to your office because her mother feels that the child's eyes turn in. The child has been healthy and seems to be progressing normally.

OBJECTIVE 1

The student should outline the initial workup of the child.
A. Vision in both eyes (child fixes and follows with both eyes indicating good vision — no amblyopia).
B. Examine the extraocular motions of both eyes (full range of motion).
C. Look for and measure any misalignment (5° esotropia).
D. Examine the retina (no evidence of tumors or congenital scars).
E. Measure the refraction of the eye (+2.00 sphere; most babies are hyperopic).

OBJECTIVE 2

The student should outline the preoperative workup.
A. Perform a standard workup for general anesthesia.
B. Be aware that a main worry is malignant hyperthermia and query the family accordingly. If there is a history, a serum creatinine phosphokinase (CPK) and, possibly, a muscle biopsy are indicated.

OBJECTIVE 3

The student should define a surgical plan that may include medical recession or resection of the lateral rectus and recession of the medial rectus muscle.

Achievement Level

OBJECTIVE 1

Minimum Level of Achievement for Passing

The student should:
A. Be able to define esotropia.
B. Describe the necessary workup.

Honors Level of Achievement

The student should:

A. Understand the relationship between strabismus and poor retinal function.
B. Define retinoblastoma and describe its presentation.

OBJECTIVE 2

Minimum Level of Achievement for Passing

The student should:

A. Understand the workup necessary for general anesthesia.
B. Know the importance of malignant hyperthermia.

Honors Level of Achievement

The student should know the histology and chemical abnormality of malignant hyperthermia.

OBJECTIVE 3

Minimum Level of Achievement for Passing

The student should understand the basic mechanics of esotropia.

Honors Level of Achievement

The student should understand the different surgical approaches and the reasons behind them.

4 Plastic Surgery: Diseases of the Skin and Soft Tissue, Face, and Hand

Case 1

You are the attending physician when a 46-year-old man is brought to the emergency room after being involved in an automobile accident as the driver. The patient appears to have struck his face in the accident and has a significant amount of facial swelling. He denies loss of consciousness.

OBJECTIVE 1

The student should recognize the possibility of injury to other areas, such as the cervical spine, globe, intracranial structures, chest, abdomen, and extremities.
  A. ABCs of resuscitation.
  B. Prioritize steps in treating the injury.
  C. Basic examination maneuvers (observation, palpation, auscultation).
  D. Further examinations necessary (electrocardiogram [ECG], x-ray).

OBJECTIVE 2

The student should outline the examination and diagnosis of facial injuries.
  A. Diagnostic examinations for potential facial injuries (physical examination, x-rays, including Water's view, computed tomography [CT] scan).
  B. Common types of facial fractures (zygomatic complex, Le Fort I, Le Fort II, Le Fort III, and mandibular).
  C. General concepts of facial fracture treatment.

Achievement Level

OBJECTIVE 1

Minimum Level of Achievement for Passing

The student:
  A. Can outline the ABCs of resuscitation.
  B. Recognizes the possibility of other injuries.
  C. Can outline an acceptable treatment plan.

Honors Level of Achievement

The student:
  A. Appropriately prioritizes treatment procedures.
  B. Recognizes the possibility of cervical spine injuries and protects the spine during further examination.

OBJECTIVE 2

Minimum Level of Achievement for Passing

The student:
  A. Recognizes the importance of physical examination followed by radiographic evaluation.
  B. Has a general understanding of the types of facial fractures.

Honors Level of Achievement

The student can correctly describe the zygomatic complex, Le Fort I, Le Fort II, and Le Fort III facial fractures.

Case 2

An 82-year-old diabetic farmer cuts his hand with a dirty shovel sustaining a deep laceration on the palmar surface. He does not come in for medical attention until the next day.

OBJECTIVE 1

The student should recognize the wound problems of diabetes, age, contamination, and delay in treatment.
  A. Problems associated with age and diabetes.
  B. Problems associated with gross contamination.
  C. Appropriate wound care for this patient.

OBJECTIVE 2

The student should describe how to do a basic hand examination.
  A. Sensory distribution of the median, ulnar, and radial nerves in the hand.
  B. Tendon examination of the hand.
  C. Vascular assessment of the hand.

Achievement Level

OBJECTIVE 1

Minimum Level of Achievement for Passing

The student should:
  A. Recognize the potential effects of age, diabetes, wound contamination, and delay in treating the wound.
  B. Describe appropriate wound care (hemostasis, irrigation, dressing, tetanus prophylaxis, antibiotics).
  C. Recognize this as a contaminated wound outside of the acceptable time for wound closure.
  D. Recognize the need for x-rays and wound culture.

Honors Level of Achievement

The student can correctly outline the adverse mechanisms in wound healing and infection caused by diabetes and delay in treatment.

OBJECTIVE 2

Minimum Level of Achievement for Passing

The student:
  A. Has a general knowledge of an appropriate examination.
  B. Can describe appropriate wound care in this situation.

Honors Level of Achievement

The student can:
  A. Demonstrate how to do a complete examination of the hand, including assessment of vascular, nerve, and tendon function.
  B. Describe the importance of Zone II lacerations.

Case 3

You are called to the newborn nursery to examine an infant with a congenital cleft deformity to the face.

OBJECTIVE 1

The student should correctly identify complete cleft lip, incomplete cleft lip, bilateral cleft lip, and cleft palate deformities.
  A. Pertinent physical findings in cleft deformity.
  B. Potential difficulties (feeding, breathing, middle ear abnormalities).

OBJECTIVE 2

The student should recognize that cleft deformities are frequently associated with other birth defects and conduct a complete physical examination of the infant.

OBJECTIVE 3

The student should recognize the importance of taking a family history and ask about a history of birth defects.

Achievement Level

OBJECTIVE 1

Minimum Level of Achievement for Passing

The student should be able to evaluate correctly deformities of the lip and palate.

Honors Level of Achievement

The student can differentiate between clefts of the primary and secondary palates.

OBJECTIVE 2

Minimum Level of Achievement for Passing

The student recognizes the possibility of other birth defects.

Honors Level of Achievement

The student recognizes other organ system abnormalities may be associated with cleft deformities.

OBJECTIVE 3

Minimum Level of Achievement for Passing

The student:
  A. Recognizes the familial tendency of cleft deformities.
  B. Can take an appropriate family history.

Honors Level of Achievement

The student can correctly counsel the parents regarding the probability of future offspring having cleft deformities.

Case 4

A 45-year-old black male presents with an ulcer on the lower extremity.

OBJECTIVE 1

The student should obtain an appropriate history.
  A. Duration of the ulcer.
  B. Prior episodes of ulceration.
  C. Location of the ulcer.
  D. Signs and symptoms (pain, numbness, infection, bleeding).
  E. Pertinent family history (sickle cell disease).
  F. Other medical history (diabetes, phlebitis).

OBJECTIVE 2

The student should outline a diagnostic plan.
  A. Physical examination.
  B. Assessment of circulation.
  C. Wound cultures.
  D. Specialized tests (noninvasive vascular studies, arteriography, complete blood count [CBC], hemoglobin electrophoresis).

OBJECTIVE 3

The student should have a basic knowledge of wound care in extremity ulcerations.
  A. Role of dressings.
  B. Role of antibiotics.
  C. Role of surgical intervention.

OBJECTIVE 4

The student should recognize that an ulcer may have more than one contributing cause.

Achievement Level

OBJECTIVE 1

Minimum Level of Achievement for Passing

The student should:
  A. Take a personal and family history.
  B. Take a history of the ulcer.

Honors Level of Achievement

The student should describe the mechanism of lower extremity ulcerations, ischemia, venous stasis, diabetes, and sickle cell disease.

OBJECTIVE 2

Minimum Level of Achievement for Passing

The student should outline an appropriate treatment plan including physical examination, assessment of circulation, and specialized studies where indicated.

Honors Level of Achievement

The student should understand the use of skin grafts and flaps in lower extremity reconstruction.

OBJECTIVE 4

Minimum Level of Achievement for Passing

The student should understand that more than one factor may be contributing to lower extremity ulcerations (venous stasis disease in a diabetic, large vessel atherosclerosis in a patient with sickle cell disease).

Honors Level of Achievement

The student should mention the possibility of malignant degeneration in a chronic ulceration.

Case 5

A 50-year-old, recently divorced female patient asks you about having a face-lift. What are the important factors in evaluating the patient?

OBJECTIVE 1

The student should recognize the importance of the physician-patient relationship.
  A. Patient's general health, skin condition, psychologic status, motivation.
  B. Factors that would discourage the patient from having the procedure.

OBJECTIVE 2

The student should identify contributing medical factors in evaluating the patient.
  A. Diabetes, hypertension.
  B. Medication history (aspirin, anticoagulants).
  C. Smoking.

Achievement Level

OBJECTIVE 1

Minimum Level of Achievement for Passing

The student should:
  A. Recognize the contributions of health, psychologic profile, and motivation.
  B. Recognize factors important in discouraging the procedure: poor motivation, unreasonable expectations, poor rapport between patient and doctor.

OBJECTIVE 2

Minimum Level of Achievement for Passing

The student recognizes the adverse effects of the following on the outcome of the procedure:

A. Some medical illnesses, such as diabetes and hypertension.
B. Some medications, such as aspirin and anticoagulants.
C. Smoking.

Honors Level of Achievement

The student presents a concise outline of the preoperative evaluation of and discussion with the patient covering all important points.

Case 6

A man falls on a branch of wood 2 days before presenting to you with a small draining wound in his left lower abdomen. The surrounding area is red, firm, and very tender. The patient has had a fever and chills for 8 hours.

OBJECTIVE

The student should recognize all the components of the injury.
A. The wound is infected.
B. The wound should not be closed.
C. Cultures should be taken.
D. Antibiotics are necessary.
E. Tetanus status should be ascertained and, if necessary, immunization and hyperimmune globulin given.
F. A foreign body may be present.
G. X-rays are necessary (to show foreign bodies, gas in the tissues).
H. Hospitalization is necessary.
I. The possibility of intraabdominal penetration should be considered.
K. The general medical status of the patient (illnesses such as diabetes) and medications he might be taking may affect the course of the infection.

Achievement Level

Minimum Level of Achievement for Passing

The student should appreciate all of the components of the injury.

Honors Level of Achievement

The student can outline all of the components in a logical fashion.

Case 7

A 65-year-old female develops a sacral decubitus ulcer. Discuss the factors affecting healing and the options for healing/reconstruction.

OBJECTIVE

The student should:
A. Recognize the importance of the patient's general medical status, emphasizing concurrent disease and medication.
B. Be able to evaluate the wound in regards to depth, infection, tissue viability, and vascularity.
C. Be able to identify the basic concepts of care of wounds containing infected or necrotic tissue.
D. Understand the basic concepts of wound healing.
E. Be able to discuss general concepts of closure, skin grafts, and flaps.

Achievement Level

Minimum Level of Achievement for Passing

The student should know the principles of wound care and healing.

Honors Level of Achievement

The student can discuss accurately the advantages and disadvantages of each type of reconstruction, giving examples of each.

Case 8

A 20-year-old male sustains a blow to the jaw in an altercation in a bar. He is brought to the emergency room with a possible mandibular fracture.

OBJECTIVE

The student should recognize the following components of the injury:
A. The importance of the preliminary examination and of airway maintenance.
B. The importance of a complete examination of the patient.
C. The importance of an intraoral examination (assessment of airway, occlusion, and possible foreign bodies).
D. The general guidelines and options in the care of mandibular fractures (reduction into occlusion; immobilization by interdental fixation, wiring, or plating).

Achievement Level

Minimum Level of Achievement for Passing

The student:
A. Should know the principles of mandibular fracture treatment.
B. Must recognize the possibility of airway compromise.

Honors Level of Achievement

The student:
A. Can systematically discuss evaluation and treatment of the facially injured patient.
B. Can discuss rational choice of immobilization techniques.
C. Can discuss the mechanism of fracture component displacement.

Case 9

A 37-year-old farmer has his right thumb avulsed. The patient and his thumb present to you in the emergency room.

OBJECTIVE

The student should be able to:
A. Realize the importance of amputation of a thumb and consider the option of replantation.
B. Discuss early wound care of the injured hand and the amputated thumb.
C. Recognize the critical time factor associated with emergent contact with a replantation surgeon.

Achievement Level

Minimal Level of Achievement for Passing

The student should understand the principles in treating a patient with an amputated thumb.

Honors Level of Achievement

The student:
A. Can discuss the effects of warm versus cold ischemia on tissue.

B. Recognizes the time factor associated with replantation.

Case 10

A factory worker presents with a 6-month history of aching pain and occasional numbness in his hands. The discomfort may even awaken him from sleep at night.

OBJECTIVE

The student should:
A. Demonstrate a general examination of the hand.
B. Recognize the possibility of a nerve compression syndrome and describe the history and physical findings of several of the most common syndromes.
C. Recognize that the problem may be located in the cervical spine, elbow, or wrist area.
D. Outline a diagnostic workup.
E. Have a general knowledge of different modalities of treatment (change in work habits, splinting, steroid injection, surgery).
G. Be aware of other potential etiologies (e.g., vascular problems, tumors).

Achievement Level

Minimum Level of Achievement for Passing

The student should understand the principles of treating a patient with a compression neuropathy.

Honors Level of Achievement

The student:
A. Can describe anatomically the common areas of compression (cubital tunnel, carpal tunnel, Guyon's canal).
B. Can describe an acceptable plan of evaluation and treatment.
C. Recognizes chronic disease syndromes.

5 Otolaryngology: Diseases of the Head and Neck

Case 1

A 6-year-old presents to the office after failing a first grade hearing screening test.

OBJECTIVE 1

The student should establish a relevant history.
- A. Duration of suspected hearing loss (3–4 months); language development (normal).
- B. History of recurrent ear infections or respiratory allergies (none known).
- C. Family history for hearing loss (negative).
- D. History of meningitis or perinatal illness (none).
- E. Snoring, mouth breathing (none).

OBJECTIVE 2

The student should elicit the following physical findings.
- A. Ear examination (dull, injected tympanic membranes, decreased mobility on pneumatoscopy).
- B. Nose (rhinitis, pale boggy mucosa).
- C. Throat (moderate postnasal drip; no tonsillar hypertrophy).

OBJECTIVE 3

The student should establish the most likely diagnosis as otitis media with effusion, but also needs to establish hearing level by audiogram and tympanogram.

OBJECTIVE 4

The student should recommend a course of antibiotics and institute medical treatment of the rhinitis and postnasal drip.

Achievement Level

Minimum Level of Achievement for Passing
The student should:

- A. Focus on the lack of risk factors for sensorineural hearing loss and establish the suspected duration of hearing loss.
- B. Diagnose otitis media with effusion, on the basis of the history and physical examination.
- C. Know to perform audiograms and tympanograms and institute antibiotic treatment.
- D. Be able to discuss indications for tubes and know ramifications of sustained hearing loss on language development.

Honors Level of Achievement

The student should be able to:
- A. Discuss the pathophysiology of eustachian tube dysfunction and its relationship to otitis media.
- B. Outline the most likely causative organisms (*Haemophilus influenzae* and diphtheroids) as well as the influence of nasal and adenoidal factors.

Case 2

A 40-year-old otherwise healthy man presents with a unilateral left-sided hearing loss of 5 months' duration.

OBJECTIVE 1

The student should establish a history of:
- A. Infections (none recently).
- B. Hearing loss (gradually progressive).
- C. Vertigo (some vague imbalance, but no true vertigo).
- D. Tinnitus (some constant high-pitched tinnitus).
- E. Other neurologic complaints (none).
- F. History of noise exposure (none).

OBJECTIVE 2

The student should elicit the following physical findings:
A. Ear examination (normal).
B. Weber and Rinne tests (Weber lateralizes to right ear; Rinne indicates better hearing when tuning fork is held near ear canal).
C. Nystagmus (none).
D. Head or neck neurologic abnormalities (none).

OBJECTIVE 3

The student should proceed right away with the appropriate tests:
A. Audiogram (reveals gradually sloping mid-frequency left-sided sensorineural hearing loss, with poor speech discrimination).
B. Tympanogram (normal).

OBJECTIVE 4

The student should be suspicious for an acoustic neuroma and should proceed with a magnetic resonance image (MRI — reveals a 2-cm cerebellopontine angle tumor consistent with an acoustic neuroma).

OBJECTIVE 5

The student should recommend surgical removal of this benign lesion for complete cure.

Achievement Level

Minimum Level of Achievement for Passing

The student should:
A. Focus on the age of the patient, the unilateral nature of the problem, the lack of noise exposure, and the lack of accompanying vertigo to become less suspicious of presbycusis, noise-induced loss, sudden hearing loss, or Meniere's disease.
B. Be highly suspicious for an acoustic neuroma.

Honors Level of Achievement

The student should:
A. Understand that a moderate-sized acoustic neuroma in a fairly young person is a surgically resectable disease, but there is risk to the facial nerve and cochlear-vestibular nerve.
B. Be aware that an acoustic neuroma is a slowly growing benign tumor.

Case 3

A 51-year-old male with six episodes of recurrent acute sinusitis in the past 8 months is referred to the otolaryngologist.

OBJECTIVE 1

The student should establish a history of:
A. Predominant symptoms (fever, headache, and teeth pain during each episode).
B. Very slow response to a 10-day antibiotic and decongestant/antihistamine treatment for each episode.
C. Seasonal variance.
D. History of allergies (currently on allergy shots).
E. Patient is between acute episodes and not currently on medications.

OBJECTIVE 2

The student should elicit the following physical findings:
A. Nose (large turbinates, drainage from each middle meati, some nasal drainage, but no septal deviation or polyps).
B. Tenderness over the medial canthi or maxilla (none).

OBJECTIVE 3

The student should be able to discuss the workup of chronic sinusitis.
A. Perform nasal endoscopy to evaluate middle meatus and any structural problems.
B. Order computed tomography (CT) scan and coronal cuts, with particular emphasis on the osteomeatal complex.

OBJECTIVE 4

The student should be able to outline treatment.
A. Initiate further medical management to include steroid nasal sprays.
B. Discuss indications for sinus surgery and the surgical options available.

Achievement Level

Minimum Level of Achievement for Passing

The student should:
A. Focus on predisposing factors to sinus disease and establish what constitutes adequate medical treatment of acute sinusitis.
B. Understand the normal clinical course for an acute sinusitis and be able to define chronic sinusitis.
C. Understand further medical treatment and list indications for surgery.

Honors Level of Achievement

The student should:
A. Be able to discuss the pathophysiology of osteomeatal complex obstruction on sinusitis and establish the influence of systemic factors.
B. Be familiar with function endoscopic sinus surgery and how it differs from traditional surgical approaches.

Case 4

A 20-year-old female presents with an increasingly sore throat and fever over the last week.

OBJECTIVE 1

The student should establish a relevant history.
  A. Antibiotics taken for sore throat (none).
  B. Fever (as high as 102°F).
  C. Swallowing difficulties (difficulty swallowing even her own saliva today).
  D. Sore throat pain (worse on the right).

OBJECTIVE 2

The student should elicit the following physical findings.
  A. Tonsils (marked right-sided peritonsillar fullness and mild tonsillitis on both sides; uvula is shifted to the left).
  B. Nose and ear examination (normal).
  C. Neck examination (2+ anterior cervical lymphadenopathy).

OBJECTIVE 3

The student should:
  A. Suspect a peritonsillar abscess.
  B. Recommend incision and drainage of the abscess followed by antibiotic coverage for treatment of *Streptococcus* and *Staphylococcus.*

Achievement Level

Minimum Level of Achievement for Passing

The student should:
  A. Focus on the severity of the sore throat and the lack of previous antibiotic treatment.
  B. Be suspicious of a peritonsillar abscess, on the basis of symptoms and clinical finding of right-sided fullness and uvular shift.
  C. Recommend that incision and drainage be carried out.

Honors Level of Achievement

The student should:
  A. Know the most likely causative organisms (β-hemolytic streptococcus).
  B. Be able to discuss the treatment of needle drainage versus a tonsillectomy.

Case 5

A 1-year-old child presents with a midline neck mass.

OBJECTIVE 1

The student should obtain pertinent additional history to include:
  A. Length of time mass has been present (since birth).
  B. Changes in size (no).
  C. Recent infections of oropharynx (no).

OBJECTIVE 2

The student should elicit the following physical findings.
  A. Location (3-cm midline, freely movable mass).
  B. Relationship to other structures (elevates with swallowing and protruding of tongue).
  C. Other neck masses (none).
  D. Oropharyngeal lesions (none).

OBJECTIVE 3

The student should be able to outline a differential diagnosis.
  A   Thyroglossal duct cyst.
  B   Dermoid cyst.
  C   Lymph node.
  D   Lipoma.
  E. Aberrant thyroid tissue.

OBJECTIVE 4

The student should outline a definitive diagnosis and treatment plan.
  A. Thyroid scan.
  B. Surgical excision to include mass, tract, midportion of hyoid bone, and tract to base of tongue.

Achievement Level

Minimum Level of Achievement for Passing

The student should:
  A. Be able to determine the likely congenital nature of the neck mass and arrive at the diagnosis of a thyroglossal duct cyst.
  B. Be able to list a differential diagnosis.
  C. Know the importance of a preoperative thyroid scan and understand indications for excision.

Honors Level of Achievement

The student should:
  A. Be able to discuss the embryology of a thyroglossal duct cyst and understand its relationship to the hyoid bone.
  B. Understand the specific surgical treatment, which must include removal of the cyst, tract, and midportion of the hyoid.

Case 6

A 3-year-old child presents to the emergency room with stridor of 6–8 hours' duration, which has become progressively worse to the point of moderate distress.

OBJECTIVE 1

The student should rapidly focus on the pertinent history.
  A. Fever today (to 102°F).
  B. Nature of stridor (inspiratory).
  C. Recent upper respiratory infection (none).
  D. Ingestion of foreign body (none known).

OBJECTIVE 2

The student should:
  A. Be highly suspicious of epiglottitis, based on the age of the patient, the sudden onset, the short duration, the inspiratory nature of the stridor, and the associated fever.
  B. Choose to perform the diagnostic study of a portable lateral neck film, since the patient is not in severe distress.
  C. Not look down the throat with a tongue blade or do anything to agitate the patient.

OBJECTIVE 3

Once the diagnosis of epiglottitis is made on the lateral neck film, the student should:

  A. Immediately institute proper treatment (take the child to the operating room and, under general anesthesia, perform laryngoscopy and intubation).
  B. Institute antibiotic coverage for *H. influenzae.*
  C. Keep the child in the ICU for postoperative care.
  D. Expect the swelling to subside and the patient to be extubated in approximately 72 hours.

Achievement Level

Minimum Level of Achievement for Passing

The student should:
  A. Perform a quick history and assessment of the airway obstruction and, based on the presentation, correctly diagnose epiglottitis.
  B. Order a lateral neck film and have child taken to the operating room for definitive diagnosis and treatment.
  C. Know not to examine the patient with a tongue blade.
  D. Be aware of *H. influenzae* as the causative agent and treat with appropriate antibiotics.

Honors Level of Achievement

The student should:
  A. Be aware of other inflammatory causes of stridor, of specific antibiotics, and of the role of β-lactamase-resistant *H. influenzae.*
  B. Understand the decision process in determining the appropriate time for extubation, and the pros and cons of performing this procedure in the ICU versus the operating room.

6 Cardiothoracic Surgery: Diseases of the Heart, Great Vessels, and Thoracic Cavity

Case 1

You are on call for the cardiothoracic service in the ICU and are asked to see a patient who underwent coronary bypass earlier in the day. His blood pressure (BP) is 90/60 mm/Hg, his pulse is 110/minutes, and his urine output is 30 mL/hr. A pulmonary artery catheter is in place.

OBJECTIVE 1

The student should ascertain that this patient is in a low cardiac output state.
  A. Note signs of low cardiac output on physical examination, examining skin turgor, temperature, and moisture.
  B. Use the pulmonary artery catheter to obtain a cardiac index (1.8 L/min/m^2).
  C. Obtain a wedge pressure (6 mm Hg).
  D. Note intake and output balance (in — 400 mL crystalloid; out — 2000 mL urine, 250 mL mediastinal drainage).

OBJECTIVE 2

The student should determine proper treatment regimen and priorities for this patient.
  A. Determine whether the patient is hypovolemic, normovolemic, or hypervolemic.
  B. Determine whether the patient is in a low cardiac output state.
  C. Treat by raising the wedge pressure with crystalloid and colloid administration (Ringer's lactate, blood, hetastarch, or plasma).

Additional Question

Alternatively, the patient's wedge pressure is 18 mm Hg, systemic vascular resistance is 1900 dyne/sec/cm^{-5}, cardiac index is 1.8 L/min/m^2, and BP is 160/90 mm Hg.
  A. What pharmacologic manipulation is appropriate? (Vasodilation and afterload reduction; the volume status is adequate and the resistance is high.)
  B. Which drugs are particularly useful in this regard? (Sodium nitroprusside and nitroglycerin, or hydralazine.)
  C. If pharmacologic manipulation is not effective, what alternative is available? (Mechanical ventricular unloading with the intraaortic balloon pump.)

Achievement Level

OBJECTIVE 1

Minimum Level of Achievement for Passing

The student should:
  A. Recognize the physical signs of low cardiac output, including pallor, cool moist skin, peripheral vasoconstriction, altered mental state, and low urine output.
  B. Use the pulmonary artery catheter to construct a set of hemodynamic parameters.

Honors Level of Achievement

The student should:
  A. Take note of the intake and output balance to supplement the hemodynamic measurements.
  B. Recognize the patient is in a negative fluid balance and therefore hypovolemic.

OBJECTIVE 2

Minimum Level of Achievement for Passing

The student should:
  A. Realize that this patient is hypovolemic and in low cardiac output.
  B. Know that fluid administration is necessary to raise the wedge pressure. Crystalloid, hetastarch, blood, or plasma may be used.

Additional Question

Minimum Level of Achievement for Passing

The student should recognize that the low cardiac output state is a congestive one with normal or high wedge pressure and hypertension. Reduction of blood pressure with afterload reduction is therefore in order.

Honors Level of Achievement

The student should:
A. Treat the patient with peripheral vasodilators such as sodium nitroprusside or nitroglycerin.
B. Recognize the failure of pharmacologic manipulation and the possibility of inserting an intraaortic balloon pump for mechanical ventricular unloading.

Case 2

A 45-year-old man presents to your general practice office with complaints of chest pain and shortness of breath with exercise. He is a smoker (40 pack-years) and has a brother who had a heart attack at the age of 49 years. The pain is occurring with less and less exertion.

OBJECTIVE 1

The student should:
A. Ascertain the nature of the pain by asking the patient to describe the character, location, and activity or exercise that provokes the pain, and what brings relief.
B. Determine the level of exercise that brings on the pain (walking uphill and walking up one flight of stairs brings on the pain, as does sitting in a chair watching TV; the pain does not awaken him at night).

OBJECTIVE 2

The student should recognize that the pain must be characterized as moderately severe and requires expeditious workup. Rest pain is often a harbinger of serious cardiac events.
A. A stress electrocardiogram should be performed (it is positive with ECG changes and chest pain).
B. Cardiac catheterization should be performed to outline the coronary anatomy (95% obstruction of the dominant right coronary artery, 85% obstruction of the left anterior descending coronary artery).

OBJECTIVE 3

The student realizes that a significant amount of myocardium is jeopardized and that revascularization may be indicated.
A. How many bypasses should be performed? (2)
B. What conduit(s) is (are) appropriate? (Mammary arteries if possible since this is a young patient and the arterial graft has a higher long-term patency.)

C. Is this operation urgent? (Rest pain and jeopardized myocardium favor early operation.)
D. Is angioplasty appropriate? (Yes, if the obstructing lesions are technically suitable.)

Achievement Level

OBJECTIVE 1

Minimum Level of Achievement for Passing

The student should begin the assessment with a history, including the nature, characterization, and severity of the chest pain, by correlating its provocation with activity levels.

Honors Level of Achievement

The student should recognize the importance of associating the pain with minimal or no exertion and recognize the urgency of this situation.

OBJECTIVE 2

Minimum Level of Achievement for Passing

The student should recognize the need for objective proof of cardiac ischemia, as evidenced by a standard ECG or stress ECG.

Honors Level of Achievement

The student should be able to discuss the methods of stress ischemia testing and the implication of the results, including ECG changes, association of chest pain with the level of work involved, and the reperfusion abnormalities associated with thallium examinations.

OBJECTIVE 3

Minimum Level of Achievement for Passing

The student should:
A. Recognize the need for complete revascularization of all vessels that can be technically bypassed.
B. Be familiar with the various conduits for coronary bypass grafting.

Honors Level of Achievement

The student should:
A. Understand that the operation is urgent because of the rest pain and the large amount of jeopardized myocardium.
B. Recognize that the internal mammary artery grafts have a higher patency rate over the long term, especially for younger patients.
C. Recognize that angioplasty may be a suitable alternative to coronary bypass in selected instances.

Case 3

You are the surgical resident on call when a 55-year-old woman presents at the emergency room with complaints of severe tearing chest pain, numbness in her legs, and feeling faint. No previous history is elicited. Physical examination demonstrates diminished femoral pulses and a diastolic murmur at the upper left sternal border.

OBJECTIVE 1

The student should outline the initial diagnostic testing designed to elicit the source of the chest pain.
  A. Complete blood count (CBC — hematocrit [Hct] 35%, white blood cells [WBC] 18,000/mm^3).
  B. ECG (left ventricular hypertrophy [LVH], otherwise normal).
  C. Chest x-ray (enlarged mediastinal shadow).
  D. BP differential (BP higher in the right arm than the left).
  E. BP (200/60 mm Hg).
  F. Urine (normal).
  G. Electrolytes (normal).
  H. Foley catheter (clear yellow urine).

OBJECTIVE 2

The student should pinpoint the diagnosis with appropriate radiologic and other tests.
  A. Echocardiogram (question of an intimal flap in the ascending aorta).
  B. CT scan of chest with contrast (intimal flap in the ascending aorta).
  C. Transesophageal echocardiogram (ascending aortic dissection by echo, both with two-dimensional echocardiography and Doppler color flow studies; mild aortic insufficiency).
  D. Aortogram (ascending aortic dissection limited to the ascending aorta).

OBJECTIVE 3

The student should outline the preoperative preparations and operative approaches for this disease.
  A. Request CBC, SMA-7, type and cross 8 units.
  B. Initiate antihypertensive therapy with a β-blocker, follow with nitroprusside to decrease the BP while awaiting surgery.
  C. Monitor with an arterial line, a Foley catheter, and perhaps a pulmonary artery catheter.
  D. Administer prophylactic antibiotics.
  E. Indicate that the patient should undergo resection and grafting of the ascending aorta with possible resuspension or replacement of the aortic valve.

Achievement Level

OBJECTIVE 1

Minimum Level of Achievement for Passing

The student should:
  A. Recognize that an abnormal chest x-ray, normal ECG, and tearing character of the pain indicate this pain is probably not cardiac ischemia.
  B. Recognize that this is a neurologic problem that may be related to vascular insufficiency of the lower extremities.

Honors Level of Achievement

The student should recognize the BP differential and note the possibility of visceral artery occlusion.

OBJECTIVE 2

Minimum Level of Achievement for Passing

The student should recognize the need to identify objectively the presence or absence of an aortic dissection by noninvasive or invasive means. CT scan and echocardiography are useful in this regard.

Honors Level of Achievement

The student should recognize the utility of noninvasive transesophageal echocardiography as a sensitive tool for the detection of ascending aortic dissection.

OBJECTIVE 3

Minimum Level of Achievement for Passing

The student should:
  A. Recognize the need to assess renal and visceral function.
  B. Recognize the need to have blood available in the operating room.
  C. Recognize the need for antibiotics in a patient who will probably receive a prosthetic vascular graft.

Honors Level of Achievement

The student should:
  A. Recognize the need to diminish the BP and the strength of left ventricular contractility to minimize the effects of the aortic dissection while awaiting operating room time.
  B. Ensure the patient recognizes that urgent operation is indicated on ascending aortic dissections because of the risk of pericardial tamponade in nonoperatively treated patients.

Case 4

You are a thoracic surgeon and a 60-year-old man has been referred to your office because of a mass detected on a chest x-ray taken for symptoms of chronic cough. Physical examination is unremarkable; he denies symptoms of cardiopulmonary disease.

OBJECTIVE 1

The student should initiate testing to determine the diagnosis of the lung mass.
A. History of cigarette smoking (30 pack-years).
B. Sputum production or hemoptysis (no).
C. Availability of old chest x-rays with which to compare the growth rate of the mass (normal chest x-ray 2 years ago).
D. CT of the chest (3-cm mass in the the midright upper lung field, a 1.5-cm mass in the right paratracheal lymph node).
E. Bronchoscopy (no lesion seen, cytology negative).
F. Percutaneous needle biopsy (positive for squamous cell carcinoma).

OBJECTIVE 2

The student should determine whether the patient is resectable for cure.
A. Comorbid conditions (no heart or kidney disease).
B. Liver enzymes, electrolytes, CBC, protime (all normal).
C. Bone scan (normal).
D. CT of the head (normal).
E. Pulmonary function studies (forced expiratory volume at 1 second [FEV_1] 1.8 L/minute — 60%, MVV 110 L/minute — 90%).

OBJECTIVE 3

The student should realize that surgical staging and resection if possible is the only chance for cure.
A. Mediastinoscopy is performed (lymph node biopsies negative for tumor).
B. Right thoracotomy is performed (right upper lobectomy and lymph node sampling reveals a T2N0M0 tumor).

Achievement Level

OBJECTIVE 1

Minimum Level of Achievement for Passing

The student should:
A. Recognize the importance of history, especially cigarette smoking, and the possible etiology of a lung mass.
B. Recognize the CT of the chest delineates a three-dimensional mass with mediastinal lymphadenopathy.
C. Recognize that a firm treatment plan depends on a tissue diagnosis and not on x-ray shadows. Bronchoscopy and needle biopsy can effect tissue diagnosis.

Honors Level of Achievement

The student should recognize the importance of old chest x-rays in determining whether the mass was present previously, what its estimated growth rate has been if present, or whether it is a new growth.

OBJECTIVE 3

Minimum Level of Achievement for Passing

The student should demonstrate knowledge that sampling the lymph nodes visible on CT scan by mediastinoscopy is essential to the staging process.

Honors Level of Achievement

The student should:
A. Demonstrate knowledge of which operation is appropriate. A lobectomy is the standard operation; wedge resection is used for small peripheral tumors in patients with compromised pulmonary function; a pneumonectomy is used when extrication of the tumor cannot be accomplished by a lesser procedure.
B. Demonstrate knowledge of the TNM staging criteria in terms of size of tumor, location of positive lymph nodes, and presence or absence of metastases.

Case 5

You are a thoracic surgeon and an 18-year-old man presents complaining of pressure in his chest, fatigue, and lassitude. A chest x-ray reveals an abnormal mediastinal contour.

OBJECTIVE 1

The student should try to establish the nature of the abnormality appearing on the chest x-ray and whether it relates to the symptoms.
A. Other symptoms (night sweats, fever, dyspnea, inguinal lymphadenopathy).
B. Masses in the scrotum (no).
C. Supraclavicular nodes (no).

OBJECTIVE 2

The student should attempt to delineate and define the abnormality in the mediastinum.
A. Posteroanterior (PA) and lateral chest x-ray to determine whether the mass is in the anterior, middle, or posterior mediastinum (anterior).

B. CT scan of the chest with contrast (the mass is anterior to the trachea).

OBJECTIVE 3

The student should arrange for preoperative testing and workup with preparation for appropriate surgical procedures.
  A. CBC, SMA-20, protime (normal).
  B. ECG (normal).
  C. Mediastinoscopy (biopsy is positive for Hodgkin's lymphoma).
  D. Biopsy of inguinal lymph nodes is performed (positive for Hodgkin's disease).
  E. CT scan of the abdomen (normal).
  F. Oncology consult for chemoradiotherapy is sought.

Achievement Level

OBJECTIVE 1

Minimum Level of Achievement for Passing

The student recognizes the signs commonly associated with malignant mediastinal masses, such as pain, dyspnea on exertion, fever, chills, and cough.

Honors Level of Achievement

The student recognizes extrathoracic sources of mediastinal masses in young men, such as testicular tumors.

OBJECTIVE 2

Minimum Level of Achievement for Passing

The student should:
  A. Attempt to assess the location of the mass by chest x-ray, since different tumors appear in the anterior, middle, and posterior mediastinum.
  B. Attempt to assess a more precise location by CT scan to determine the most successful route for biopsy via needle biopsy, mediastinoscopy, or mediastinotomy.

Honors Level of Achievement

The student should be aware that anterior mediastinal tumors are often thymoma, teratoma, and thyroid; middle mediastinal tumors are often lymph node metastases and lymphoma; posterior mediastinal tumors are often neurogenic.

Case 6

You are the surgical resident on call when a 65-year-old woman presents to the emergency room with a history of coughing up blood for the past 12 hours. Apparently, she has filled two saucepans at home with blood. There is no history of previous lung disease.

OBJECTIVE 1

The student should try to establish the etiology and severity of the hemoptysis.
  A. CBC (Hct 31%, WBC 18,000/mm^3).
  B. Arterial blood gases (pH 7.47, PCO$_2$ 28 mm Hg, PCO$_2$ 62 mm Hg, 88% saturated).
  C. Chest x-ray (infiltrate in left upper lobe).
  D. Patient has a history of heavy smoking but no chest pain or previous shortness of breath.

OBJECTIVE 2

The student should realize early definitive diagnosis and lateralization is mandatory because the hemoptysis has caused significant blood loss and is interfering with oxygenation.

Perform early flexible bronchoscopy (blood is noted to be coming from the left main stem bronchus; the tumor mass is seen inside the left upper lobe orifice obstructing it by 90%).

OBJECTIVE 3

The student should initiate treatment for hemoptysis.
  A. Humidified oxygen.
  B. Morphine sulfate for sedation.
  C. Codeine as an antitussive.
  D. Broad-spectrum antibiotics.
  E. Bed rest.
  F. Left side down at all times.

Additional Question

Massive hemoptysis recurs despite conservative measures.
  1. What is the next maneuver? (Repeat rigid bronchoscopy.)
  2. What means can be used to stop the bleeding? [(a) Balloon blockade; (b) a double-lumen endobronchial catheter; (c) yittrium aluminum garnert (YAG) laser bronchoscopy, and (d) bronchial artery arteriography with embolization.]

Achievement Level

OBJECTIVES 1 AND 2

Minimum Level of Achievement for Passing

The student should:
  A. Realize that the Hct and Hgb level will reflect the amount of blood lost.
  B. Realize that blood gases will assess the effect on ventilation and oxygenation and will indicate if hypoxemia is present despite hyperventilation.
  C. Realize that a chest x-ray will help lateralize the source of the bleeding, so that if emergency thoracotomy is necessary, proper treatment can be initiated.

Honors Level of Achievement

The student recognizes that early bronchoscopy will definitively lateralize the source of the bleeding for future treatment and may also confirm the etiology of the hemoptysis. Waiting until bleeding stops may preclude establishment of diagnosis and the ability to lateralize the process.

OBJECTIVE 3

Minimum Level of Achievement for Passing

The student recognizes that massive hemoptysis is due to inflammatory diseases in most instances; oxygen, humidity, antibiotics, antitussives, and bed rest are therefore indicated.

Additional Question

Honors Level of Achievement

Emergency treatment for massive hemoptysis includes bronchoscopy with balloon blockade, double-lumen catheters, laser use, and embolization.

Case 7

You are the surgical resident on call when a 45-year-old man presents in the emergency room because of fever, lethargy, and foul-smelling, purulent sputum production of 1 week's duration. He has not eaten for 3 days.

OBJECTIVE 1

The student should ascertain the nature of the pathology of the respiratory system.
  A. Physical history (prior history of respiratory illness, nature of illness, nature of the sputum, length of current illness).
  B. Social history (alcoholism — yes; cigarette smoking — yes; living conditions — lives alone).
  C. Physical examination, listening particularly to the chest and examining the head and neck area (rhonchi over the right midlung field posteriorly; no nuchal rigidity; patient appears emaciated and dehydrated; temperature is 40.1°C rectally).
  D. CBC (Hgb 8.3 g/dL, Hct 25%, WBC 22,000/mm^3 with shift to the left); electrolytes (blood urea nitrogen [BUN] 42 mg/dL, otherwise normal).
  E. Sputum sample (numerous WBCs, too many Gram-positive rods to count; foul odor).
  F. Chest x-ray (PA — large cavity with an air fluid level in the right midlung field; lateral — cavity appears posteriorly at the level of T-4 to T-8).

OBJECTIVE 2

The student, recognizing the presence of a lung abscess, should take steps to ascertain the etiology and initiate therapy.
  A. History of blacking out, fainting, falling, or stupor (patient cannot remember the last 3 days).
  B. Evidence of endobronchial obstruction (flexible bronchoscopy reveals edema and purulence at the orifice of the superior segment of the right lower lobe but shows no endobronchial masses).
  C. Attempt to drain abscess (bronchoscope is passed into the superior segment in effort to drain purulence; deep cultures are obtained as well).
  D. Attempt to use gravity to drain abscess (postural drainage and chest physiotherapy are encouraged to promote drainage).
  E. Decision on antibiotic coverage (Gram stain demonstrates Gram-positive rods; therapy is initiated with broad-spectrum antibiotics that cover Gram-negative and Gram-positive organisms until cultures are available; penicillin, 3–20 million units daily, and aminoglycoside are begun i.v.).

OBJECTIVE 3

The student should recognize failure of the current therapy to resolve the septic state and describe other possible therapeutic measures.
  A. Inadequate drainage of the cavity (chest x-ray confirms the continued presence of an air fluid level).
  B. Cavity amenable to other forms of drainage (CT scan confirms the cavity is in continuity with the chest wall).
  C. Percutaneous tube drainage of the abscess (air fluid level disappears).
  D. Long-term treatment of this patient (most abscess cavities resolve with drainage and continued antibiotics; occasionally, pulmonary resection is indicated after the septic state has resolved and the patient's debilitative condition is reversed).

Achievement Level

OBJECTIVE 1

Minimum Level of Achievement for Passing

The student should:
  A. Recognize some of the historical features that predispose patients to aspiration and lung abscess.
  B. Order a chest x-ray to delineate the nature of the pulmonary pathology.

Honors Level of Achievement

The student should examine the Gram stain of the sputum to begin appropriate antibiotic therapy before obtaining results of cultures, which may take 24–48 hours.

OBJECTIVE 2

Minimum Level of Achievement for Passing

The student should recognize the need for examination of the bronchial tree endoscopically to rule out endobronchial obstruction as a cause of the infection and abscess.

Honors Level of Achievement

The student should know to apply endoscopic drainage in an effort to promote resolution of the abscessed cavity.

OBJECTIVE 3

Minimum Level of Achievement for Passing

The student should:
  A. Recognize the failure of antibiotic and endoscopic therapy by virtue of the continued presence of an air fluid level on chest x-ray.
  B. Recognize the need to promote better drainage in this patient.

Honors Level of Achievement

The student should know to attempt percutaneous tube thoracostomy in patients with an abscessed lung cavity who are too sick to undergo thoracotomy and resection.

Case 8

You are a thoracic surgeon in private practice and a 60-year-old woman presents at your office complaining of left-sided chest pain, fever, weakness, anorexia, and weight loss for the past 6 weeks.

OBJECTIVE 1

The student should elucidate pertinent historical information to determine the etiology of the complaint.
  A. Symptoms (pain exacerbated by a deep breath; sputum with a foul odor is produced when patient lying down; no hemoptysis).
  B. Previous respiratory illnesses (history of tuberculosis exposure years ago for which she took two pills daily for 1 year; skin test reported positive at that time).
  C. Physical examination to ascertain metabolic and nutritional state of the patient and to note chest sounds and movement (patient appears emaciated, her tongue is dry, skin turgor poor, eyes sunken; coarse rales in all lung fields, but markedly diminished breath sounds on the left side, not as much movement of the chest wall on the left as on the right side, percussion note dull on left and normal on right side).
  D. Chest x-ray (hazy opacification of the entire left hemithorax; mediastinum and heart appear to be shifted to the right).
  E. CBC (Hct 42%, WBC 17,500/mm^3 with marked shift to the left).
  F. Electrolytes and SMA examination (normal except for BUN 56 mg/dL, elevated liver transaminase, and albumin 1.9 g/dL).
  G. Thoracentesis (reveals foul, purulent fluid).
  H. Gram stain immediately before culturing (reveals many white blood cells and Gram-negative rods).

OBJECTIVE 2

The student should recognize the presence of a pleural empyema and begin treatment.
  A. Insert large-bore test tube (yields 2400 ml of murky, foul-smelling fluid).
  B. Repeat chest x-ray (small air fluid level remains at the base, and the lung is incompletely expanded, showing 2- to 3-cm rind around the left lung).
  C. Observe patient clinically over the next 24–48 hours (patient remains febrile with chest pain and mild shortness of breath).
  D. Assure adequate nutritional intake either i.v. or by mouth (p.o.).

The patient remains clinically infected with fever, night sweats, anorexia, and elevated white count.

OBJECTIVE 3

The student should consider the most effective way of resolving the fact that the lung is not fully expanded and the pleural space remains infected.
  A. Rib resection and drainage of the pleural space (this option rejected since it appears that the fluid is draining but the lung is trapped within the pleural space).
  B. Thoracotomy and decortication (the rind around the lung is removed, the lung is fully expanded, and the pleural space obliterated by appropriate tube drainage).

Achievement Level

OBJECTIVE 1

Minimum Level of Achievement for Passing

The student should:
  A. Obtain appropriate historical information leading to the discovery of the patient's probable tuberculosis exposure many years ago, and therefore the potential for pleuropulmonary disease.

B. Elicit the physical findings suggestive of fluid in the pleural space and severe dehydration and malnutrition.

Honors Level of Achievement

The student should recognize that the opacification on the chest x-ray represents fluid rather than atelectasis and decides to pursue thoracentesis because of the fact that the mediastinum is shifted contralaterally.

OBJECTIVE 2

Minimum Level of Achievement for Passing

The student should:
A. Sample the fluid to ascertain the presence and nature of the infection.
B. Immediately test the fluid with Gram stain to provide initial antibiotic coverage based on the organisms present.

OBJECTIVE 3

Minimum Level of Achievement for Passing

The student should obtain a repeat chest x-ray to assess the efficacy of the tube thoracostomy.

Honors Level of Achievement

The student recognizes the failure of tube thoracostomy and the presence of a trapped lung requiring decortication rather than an additional tube.

Case 9

A 4-year-old child is brought to your office because of fatigue, low growth, and bluish discoloration of the lips. His BP is 80/60 mm Hg and his pulse is 110/minutes.

OBJECTIVE 1

The student should obtain historical information pertinent to narrowing the diagnosis.
A. Normal birth (yes).
B. Hospitalizations (none).
C. Episodes of wheezing and shortness of breath (only when crying).
D. Squatting (yes).
E. Fatigue (yes).
F. Percentage growth curve (43% by the pediatrician).
G. "Spelling" (yes).

OBJECTIVE 2

The student should conduct pertinent physical examination tests to narrow the diagnosis.
A. Color of lips (blue).

B. Clubbing of fingers and toes (yes).
C. Palpation of the chest (a harsh thrill at the left sternal border).
D. Auscultation of the heart (3/6 systolic ejection murmur at the upper left sternal border).
E. Murmur decreases when the baby is crying and grunting (yes).

OBJECTIVE 3

The student should obtain objective information about the diagnosis.
A. Hgb (21 g/dL) and Hct (65%).
B. Bleeding time (14 minutes).
C. Chest x-ray (decreased pulmonary vasculature and a "coeur en sabot").
D. ECG (right ventricular hypertrophy).
E. Echocardiogram (an overriding aorta and a subaortic ventricular septal defect [VSD]).
F. Catheterization (equal pressures in the left and right ventricles, normal coronary arteries, and a right-sided aortic arch).

OBJECTIVE 4

The student should be able to narrow the diagnosis.
A. Congenital heart disease (yes).
B. Acyanotic heart disease (no).
C. Cyanotic heart disease (yes).
D. Left-to-right shunt (no).
E. Right-to-left shunt (yes).
F. Truncus arteriosus (no).
G. Tetralogy of Fallot (yes).
H. Transposition of the great arteries (no).

Additional Questions

You have determined that the diagnosis is tetralogy of Fallot. Preoperative considerations important to designing an operative procedure include:
1. What is the blood type? (AB+).
2. What side would a Blalock-Taussig shunt be on? (left) Why? (opposite the aortic arch).
3. What are the main considerations for total repair? (age and pulmonary artery size).
4. What are the principles of total repair? (closure of the VSD and opening the right ventricular outflow tract so that the right-sided pressures are 2/3 systemic or less).

Achievement Level

OBJECTIVE 1

Minimum Level of Achievement for Passing

The student should recognize the physical signs of cyanotic congenital heart disease.

Honors Level of Achievement

The student should recognize squatting and spelling as being typical signs for tetralogy of Fallot.

OBJECTIVE 2

Minimum Level of Achievement for Passing

The student should note in the physical examination the lip color, clubbing, and characteristics of the heart murmur.

Honors Level of Achievement

The student should recognize the decrease in the heart murmur when the patient performs a Valsalva maneuver or is crying.

OBJECTIVE 3

Minimum Level of Achievement for Passing

The student should:
   A. Recognize the markedly increased Hct and Hgb with cyanotic congenital heart disease.
   B. Recognize the right ventricular hypertrophy and the echocardiographic findings of subaortic VSD and pulmonic stenosis.

Honors Level of Achievement

The student should recognize the decreased pulmonary vasculature on the chest x-ray, the equalization of the pressures in the right and left ventricles, and the right-sided aortic arch as typical of tetralogy of Fallot.

OBJECTIVE 4

Minimum Level of Achievement for Passing

The student should recognize this patient has cyanotic congenital heart disease.

Honors Level of Achievement

The student should recognize that the patient has a right-to-left shunt representing tetralogy of Fallot, not transposition of the great arteries.

Additional Questions

Minimum Level of Achievement for Passing

The student should recognize that the criteria for repair include patient age and pulmonary artery size.

Honors Level of Achievement

The student should:
   A. Recognize the side of the Blalock-Taussig shunt referable to the aortic arch.
   B. Recognize that the principles of repair include VSD closure and enlargement of the right ventricular outflow tract.

7 Orthopedics: Diseases of the Musculoskeletal System

Case 1

You are the orthopedic resident on duty and are called to the emergency room to evaluate a 65-year-old female who presents with a deformed right wrist after slipping on the ice and falling on the outstretched hand.

OBJECTIVE 1

The student should be able to elicit the history noting:
  A. Length of time since the fall, any symptoms of neurovascular compromise, any attempts by patient or others at reduction of the deformity.
  B. Pertinent past medical history (allergies, medications, previous fractures, past surgical procedures, response to anesthetic, review of systems).
  C. Hand dominance and occupation of patient.

OBJECTIVE 2

The student should be able to describe the following regarding a Colles' fracture.
  A. Clinical appearance (dorsal displacement, radial deviation, and angulation with dorsal fragment angled dorsally or apex volar; assessment of neurovascular integrity; open or closed injury).
  B. Radiographic assessment (level of fracture; plus involvement of articular surface; direction and amount of displacement; direction and degree of angulation; impaction and shortening; and involvement of carpal bones, i.e., associated scaphoid fracture or lunate dislocation).

OBJECTIVE 3

The student should be able to describe the management of an uncomplicated Colles' fracture.
  A. Reduction after appropriate local, regional, or general anesthetic; traction in the line of deformity; disimpaction of the fragments; manipulation to correct the deformity.
  B. Cast immobilization.
  C. Rehabilitation of function after the fracture has healed and the cast has been removed.

Achievement Level

OBJECTIVE 1

Minimum Level of Achievement for Passing

The student should obtain a history, including mechanism of injury, time from injury to present, symptoms suggesting neurovascular compromise, pertinent past medical history.

Honors Level of Achievement

The student should inquire about attempts at reduction, response to previous anesthetics, hand dominance, and occupation.

OBJECTIVE 2

Minimum Level of Achievement for Passing

The student should:
  A. Describe the clinical appearance of a typical Colles' fracture (dorsal displacement and angulation, radial deviation).
  B. Describe the basic radiologic features of a typical Colles' fracture (fracture of the distal radius, direction and amount displacement, degree of angulation).

Honors Level of Achievement

The student should:
  A. Assess the integrity of the distal neurovascular system (color, temperature, capillary filling, sensation, attempt at motor examination including integrity of long flexor tendons) and whether injury is closed or open.
  B. Assess intraarticular involvement and possible associated carpal injuries.

OBJECTIVE 3

Minimum Level of Achievement for Passing

The student should be able to relate the usual accepted method of Colles' fracture treatment including reduction, immobilization, and rehabilitation.

Honors Level of Achievement

The student should:
A. Consider the type of anesthetic used.
B. Describe appropriate methods of traction and closed reduction.
C. Show awareness of the propensity for the reduction not to be maintained and suggest methods used to maintain the reduction (K wire fixation).
D. Following reduction and immobilization, reassess the neurovascular function.

Case 2

As the orthopedic consultant in the emergency room, you are asked to see a 21-year-old male who has an obvious open fracture of the right tibia: the broken bone is visible in the wound over the anterior aspect of the tibia. You are assured by the general surgeon in charge of the trauma team that there are no other associated injuries and the patient is hemodynamically stable.

OBJECTIVE 1

The student should outline pertinent features of the history.
A. Time of accident.
B. Mechanism of injury.
C. Site of accident and possible contaminating factors.
D. History from ambulance personnel (position of the leg, whether bone was protruding, estimated blood loss prior to arrival, what was done by ambulance personnel prior to arrival).
E. Past history (medications, allergies, status regarding tetanus prophylaxis).

OBJECTIVE 2

In an orderly fashion, the student should:
A. Check the neurovascular status of the extremity.
B. Splint the extremity if not already done.

C. Culture the wound and cover with a sterile dressing.
D. Commence appropriate antibiotic coverage.
E. Administer appropriate tetanus prophylaxis.
F. Obtain anteroposterior (AP) and lateral radiographs of the injured extremity, including appropriate radiographs of the joint above and the joint below.
G. Prepare the patient for a general anesthetic in the operating room, performing the standard laboratory investigations and assuring that the cross-match has been made.
H. Take the patient to the operating room and under sterile conditions prepare and drape the extremity and carry out appropriate debridement and irrigation.
I. After the wound is as clean as possible, reprepare and redrape and, with a new set of instruments, perform reduction and immobilization appropriately.
J. Leave the wound open.

Achievement Level

OBJECTIVE 1

Minimum Level of Achievement for Passing

The student should outline essential features of the history, including time of injury, site, and mechanism of injury.

Honors Level of Achievement

The student should additionally discuss information obtained from the ambulance personnel and show understanding that the site of accident may be important in determining possible contaminating organisms, such as clostridial contamination in farm injuries.

OBJECTIVE 2

Minimum Level of Achievement for Passing

The student should assess the neurovascular status, culture the wound, commence antibiotic and tetanus prophylactic coverage, obtain radiographs of the lower leg, and proceed to the operating room for debridement, irrigation, and reduction. The wound should be left open.

Honors Level of Achievement

The student should note that radiographs of the joint above and the joint below must be taken, that the patient should be prepared for general anesthetic, and that cross-match must be done. When discussing forms of immobilization, the student should mention that in open fractures internal fixation is usually contraindicated and that the wound should be left open.

Case 3

As the orthopedic resident on duty, you are called by the nurse in charge of the orthopedic ward requesting an increase in narcotic analgesia for a patient admitted 6 hours ago following a closed reduction of a tibia/fibula fracture and immobilization in an above-knee cast.

OBJECTIVE 1

The student should be able to discuss the possibility of a compartment syndrome developing after closed reductions and plaster immobilization.

OBJECTIVE 2

The student should assess the neurovascular status of the extremity and the response to passive stretching of the muscles in the suspected compartment. If symptoms and signs suggest a compartment syndrome, the cast must be split to the skin. If symptoms and signs are not relieved, then the cast must be removed, compartment pressures measured, and open fasciotomy considered.

Achievement Level

OBJECTIVE 1

Minimum Level of Achievement for Passing

The student should consider the possibility of a compartment syndrome and not merely give a verbal order for increased analgesia.

Honors Level of Achievement

The student should ask the nurse:
  A. Time since and amount of last dose of analgesia.
  B. Status of the neurovascular examination of the exposed foot.

OBJECTIVE 2

Minimum Level of Achievement for Passing

The student should examine the patient and assess the degree of pain, color, and temperature of the exposed distal extremity; sensory and motor function; response to passive stretching of the flexors and extensors of the toes. If a compartment syndrome is suggested, open fasciotomy must be carried out.

Honors Level of Achievement

The student should relate that the presence of pulses does not rule out a compartment syndrome and that intracompartmental pressure measurements comparing with the normal opposite extremity are the most important criteria for diagnosing a compartment syndrome.

Case 4

As the orthopedic resident on call, you are asked to assess a 21-year-old male in the emergency room who has fallen while skating and complains of right shoulder pain.

OBJECTIVE 1

The student should:
  A. Elicit the history, including mechanism of injury, time of injury, location of pain, radiation of pain, nature of pain, symptoms suggesting neurovascular involvement.
  B. Ask about previous episodes related to the same shoulder.

OBJECTIVE 2

The student should relate an orderly physical examination, including:
  A. Observation and comparison with the opposite shoulder; presence or absence of deformity.
  B. Palpation of deformity; localization of maximal tenderness.
  C. No attempt at active or passive motion if dislocation or fracture is suspected.
  D. Assess neurovascular status.

OBJECTIVE 3

The student should be able to give a differential diagnosis including dislocation of the shoulder, acromioclavicular joint injury, and fracture of the proximal humerus.

Achievement Level

Minimum Level of Achievement for Passing

The student should:
  A. Illustrate the ability to elicit an adequate history regarding musculoskeletal injuries, including the mechanism of injury; the time of injury; and description of pain according to location, radiation, and type.
  B. Be able to relate an orderly physical examination of the injured extremity, including inspection, palpation, range of motion, and neurovascular assessment.
  C. Be able to describe the physical and radiologic findings with anterior and posterior dislocation of the shoulder.
  D. Consider in the differential diagnosis shoulder dislocation, fracture, and acromioclavicular joint injury.

Honors Level of Achievement

The student should:

A. Consider history related to neurovascular symptoms and cervical spine problems. On examination, the student should examine the cervical spine as well as the upper extremity and consider the cervical spine causes in the differential diagnosis of shoulder pain following trauma.

B. Be able to describe the findings associated with axillary nerve injury.

Case 5

A 65-year-old male presents to your office with a chief complaint of pain in the groin region. He has been told that the pain is caused by arthritis of the hip.

OBJECTIVE 1

The student should elicit on history taking the positive findings related to the hip and point out the pertinent negative findings.

A. Chief complaint: duration, location, radiation, nature of the pain; alleviating or aggravating factors.

B. Level of function of the patient.

C. Previous treatment and response to it.

OBJECTIVE 2

The student should be able to describe the findings on physical examination with moderate unilateral osteoarthritis of the hip (gait abnormalities, range of motion) and also indicate that full examination of the spine, knee, and associated neurovascular examination has been carried out.

OBJECTIVE 3

The student should be able to discuss the radiologic features of osteoarthritis of the hip (joint space narrowing, subchondral sclerosis, osteophyte formation, subchondral cyst formation).

OBJECTIVE 4

The student should:

A. Describe a conservative regimen of management (antiinflammatory medications, physiotherapy to maintain range of motion and maintain strength of muscles about the affected joint, the use of a cane in the opposite extremity, and weight reduction).

B. Describe surgical options available if a conservative regimen fails (arthroplasty, osteotomy, arthrodesis).

Achievement Level

Minimum Level of Achievement for Passing

The student should:

A. Exhibit the ability to take an adequate history regarding an arthritic joint and relate the physical and radiologic findings that would be expected in a patient with osteoarthritis of the hip.

B. Be able to discuss the conservative and surgical management of a patient that has osteoarthritis in only one hip.

Honors Level of Achievement

The student should:

A. Inquire about the functional level of the patient.

B. Ascertain response, if any, to treatment.

C. On physical examination, note factors that localize the problem to the hip joint and rule out other causes (local groin, back, intraabdominal, or pelvic pathology).

D. Know the gait abnormalities associated with osteoarthritis of the hip and the first motion usually lost in early osteoarthritis of the hip (internal rotation).

E. Be able to discuss the pros and cons of each of the surgical options in relation to the case presented.

Case 6

A 35-year-old male presents to the emergency room with a 12-hour history of acute pain and swelling in the right knee. The patient sustained a laceration of the ipsilateral foot 3 days ago that had not been treated.

OBJECTIVE 1

The student should assess the clinical features (symptoms and signs) compatible with acute septic arthritis of the knee, including:

A. Evidence of systemic illness (fever and tachycardia).

B. Redness of the joint.

C. Increased temperature of the joint.

D. Diffuse tenderness to palpation.

E. Evidence of effusion in the joint.

F. A severe limp or inability to bear weight.

G. The knee held in a partially flexed position.

H. Markedly reduced or absent range of motion, either actively or passively.

OBJECTIVE 2

The clinical diagnosis is acute septic arthritis, and the student should perform the following:

A. Obtain CBC and differential.
B. Determine sedimentation rate.
C. Culture the foot wound.
D. Do blood cultures.
E. Request plain radiographs of the knee.
F. Request bone and gallium scan.
G. Aspirate joint and do Gram stain and culture of the fluid obtained.

Achievement Level

OBJECTIVE 1

Minimum Level of Achievement for Passing

The student should be able to cite five of eight clinical features associated with septic arthritis of a joint.

Honors Level of Achievement

The student should cite seven or eight of eight clinical features.

OBJECTIVE 2

Minimum Level of Achievement for Passing

The student should perform an aspiration, Gram stain, and culture.

Honors Level of Achievement

The student should suggest six or more of eight tests listed and be able to discuss the usefulness and limitations of each test.

8 Neurosurgery: Diseases of the Central and Peripheral Nervous System

Case 1

As the neurosurgeon resident on call, you are asked to see a male in his late 50s or early 60s who was brought unconscious to the emergency room following an automobile accident that occurred 2 hours ago. The patient had to be extricated from the car. After initial examination and resuscitation, vital signs demonstrated a pulse of 100/minute, blood pressure (BP) of 115/70 mm Hg, a respiratory rate of 16/minute, and a temperature of 37.7°C. [The examiner can choose to cover all objectives, just 1–7, 8–9, 10–12, or some combination of these.]

OBJECTIVE 1

The student should perform a primary survey.
- A. Inspection of the airway (appears adequate).
- B. BP, taken by cuff (stable upon repeated measurement).
- C. Evaluation of i.v. access (reveals that no. 18 gauge i.v. has been placed).
- D. Initial neurologic examination (reveals an unconscious patient, not intubated, who becomes easily agitated moving all four extremities randomly upon tactile stimulation. The Glasgow coma score is 6. There is contusion about the right eye. The right pupil is 5 mm, the left pupil is 3 mm).

OBJECTIVE 2

The student should describe preparatory management and additional appropriate diagnostic tests to be done before therapy.

OBJECTIVE 3

The student should provide a differential diagnosis of the neurologic problem and rate its urgency.

OBJECTIVE 4

Before further diagnostic measures (which might take up to 30 minutes and require moving the patient, the student should provide initial therapy based upon the clinical picture and the laboratory results in the context of the possible neurosurgical problems. Assume that no matched blood is available for 1 hour and the patient remains normotensive.
- A. Initial x-rays (skull x-ray shows a linear right frontal fracture that passes into the frontal sinus and cervical spine x-ray shows osteoarthritic changes with good visualization to C-7).
- B. Initial blood tests (hematocrit [Hct] 35%, white blood cell [WBC] 14,300/mm^3, PO$_2$ 99 mm Hg, PCO$_2$ 48 mm Hg, no significant electrolyte imbalance, blood alcohol 150 mg/dL).

OBJECTIVE 5

Based upon the differential diagnosis of the neurologic picture, the student should order further diagnostic tests. Computed tomography (CT) scan (demonstrates a 0.5-cm thick frontal subdural hemorrhage and hemorrhagic contusion of the right frontal lobe with a shift of the midline structures; student should be able to describe the clinical signs of such an intracranial mass that might indicate compromise of brain function and threaten life).

OBJECTIVE 6

An abdominal tap performed by the general surgery team is positive for blood. The student should describe and prioritize the treatment of the neurologic injury with respect to the other known injuries and describe the measures necessary to ensure a safe removal of the intracranial pathology.

OBJECTIVE 7

Postoperatively, the pupils are equal. The patient is agitated and moves his left side less than his right. Over the first 24 hours his intracranial pressure (ICP) slowly rises from 8 to 19 mm Hg. The student should describe the possible causes and the means to control ICP elevation.

OBJECTIVE 8

The patient responds well to this regimen, and after 5 days, the ICP is less than 10 mm Hg. The ICP monitor is removed. The patient becomes more lucid, follows commands, has equal reactive pupils and normal extremity movement. The endotracheal tube is removed, but he requires a good deal of suctioning and pulmonary physiotherapy. After one such treatment, he develops weakness in all extremities. The student should reevaluate the situation by:

- A. Performing a physical examination (reveals weakness of the legs and arms sparing the deltoids, patchy loss of pin and touch perception in the extremities and in the trunk below the nipples, absent biceps reflexes but normal triceps reflexes with mild hyperreflexia at the knees and ankles, and reappearance of Babinski's sign).
- B. Arriving at a tentative diagnosis for the cause of these findings.
- C. Ordering appropriate radiologic studies.

OBJECTIVE 9

Lateral cervical spine films reveal a step-off of 5 mm between C-5 and C-6 and locking of the facets. The student should discuss the management of this problem by:

- A. Ordering additional appropriate radiologic studies (CT shows narrowing of the spinal canal and discloses facet dislocation and bilateral fractures of the C-5 lamina; magnetic resonance imaging (MRI) shows narrowing of the canal and increased T2 signal in the spinal cord at C-6).
- B. Commenting upon the available therapeutic options.

OBJECTIVE 10

Ten days after injury, the patient has a fever of 39.2°C. He is more obtunded. The student should:

- A. Perform a physical examination (reveals a temperature of 39.0°C and increased obtundation).
- B. Offer a differential diagnosis.
- C. Perform a CT scan.
- D. Perform a lumbar puncture (which yields cloudy fluid with WBC 600/mm^3, polymorphonucleated WBCs [polys] 80%, lymphocytes [lymphs] 20%, total protein 215 g/dL, glucose 43 mg/dL; Gram stain is negative).
- E. Offer a diagnosis and outline treatment.

OBJECTIVE 11

After 2 weeks of successful treatment with i.v. antibiotics, the patient stabilizes and becomes more responsive. He obeys simple commands. Clear nasal drainage has become apparent and continues to persist 1 week after treatment has been completed. The student should arrive at a preliminary diagnosis and make recommendations for further diagnostic and therapeutic measures by:

- A. Determining the origin of the nasal drainage (glucose 50 mg/dL, radioactivity elevated in

drainage following isotope cisternogram).
- B. Choosing appropriate tests to localize the site of leakage (radioactive scan demonstrates site of leakage 6 hours following instillation of isotope into the lumbar subarachnoid space; CT scan demonstrates site of leakage 4 hours after instillation of contrast media into the lumbar cerebrospinal fluid [CSF]).
- C. Recommending treatment.

OBJECTIVE 12

After further treatment, the patient is discharged to a rehabilitation unit. Medications include antiepileptic drugs. He progresses well for 2 weeks and then regresses. He becomes less cooperative, more agitated, and lethargic. His gait deteriorates again. He is referred back to your clinic.

- A. The student should provide a differential diagnosis.
- B. The student should order laboratory tests to differentiate these diagnoses.
- C. The student should be able to discuss the necessary treatment.

Achievement Level

OBJECTIVE 1

Minimum Level of Achievement for Passing

The student should:

- A. Emphasize maintenance of the airway and recognize the role of hypoxia in worsening the outcome in head trauma victims. The student should also recognize the need to assess cervical spine stability and discuss the various techniques available to secure an airway in the presence of a possible unstable cervical spine injury. Nasotracheal airway with in-line traction is preferred.
- B. Know of the need to monitor and maintain adequate BP in the setting of head trauma and be aware that in severe head trauma autoregulation is lost and cerebral perfusion depends upon mean arterial blood pressure.
- C. Know the three types of neurologic function evaluated to determine the Glasgow coma score (eye opening, motor response, verbal response) and the significance of pupillary inequality as well as disconjugate gaze.

Honors Level of Achievement

The student should be able to outline the entire Glasgow coma scale.

OBJECTIVE 2

Minimum Level of Achievement for Passing

The student should:

- A. Arrange for placement of an arterial line, a large-bore i.v. (slow infusion), and a Foley catheter.

B. Order a lateral cervical spine and a lateral skull x-ray.

C. Ask for blood tests with a particular emphasis upon the Hct, clotting studies, and blood gases, as well as electrolytes, and ascertain that blood has been sent to the blood bank for type and cross-match.

Honors Level of Achievement

The student should:

A. Recognize the need to visualize the cervical spine on a lateral film down to include the level of T-1 and describe how this may be achieved.

B. List the skull x-ray findings that raise the possibility of basilar skull fractures (intracranial air).

OBJECTIVE 3

Minimum Level of Achievement for Passing

The student should:

A. Provide the differential diagnosis for the cause of the neurologic findings with closed head trauma, including alcohol intoxication, cerebral contusion, axonal shearing, intracerebral subdural and/or epidural hematoma, and local trauma to the eye. The student should explain the likelihood that alcoholic intoxication is the only cause of the patient's condition.

B. Offer a level of urgency of the neurosurgical problem and explain why this level of urgency is being considered.

OBJECTIVE 4

The student should:

A. Recognize the need to immobilize the neck as soon as possible, especially before intubation or other maneuvers, and list methods of immobilizing the neck (collar, tongs, manual traction, halo).

B. Recognize that the hypercarbia requires correction and discuss why this is so and how it is to be accomplished.

C. Offer a detailed discussion of the immediate and longer term fluid management of the head injury and anemia; address the need to combine management of blood loss and ICP elevation; address the need to locate the source of blood loss and the likelihood that it arises from intracranial bleeding.

OBJECTIVE 5

The student should:

A. Order a CT scan as soon as possible, list the indications for immediate CT scanning of this patient, and describe what might be done if CT is not available.

B. Describe the signs of progressive transtentorial herniation, including pupillary, motor, and respiratory changes.

Honors Level of Achievement

The student should:

A. Describe the CT findings with intracerebral hematoma, cerebral contusion with edema, acute subdural hematoma, and epidural hematoma.

B. Describe the anatomical structures involved and the pathology caused by transtentorial herniation.

OBJECTIVE 6

The student should:

A. Recognize that craniotomy with removal of the subdural hematoma and possibly of contused brain is necessary.

B. Recognize that the surgical removal of the intracranial mass cannot wait until laparotomy has been completed, but that laparotomy for bleeding must also be done emergently and, hence, concurrently with craniotomy.

C. Plan to insert an ICP monitor, either pre- or postoperatively, discuss the role of ICP monitoring, and state the normal level of ICP (under 15 mm Hg).

Honors Level of Achievement

The student should:

A. List the important determinants of prognosis in cases of severe head injury.

B. Be able to name the different means of ICP measurement and describe their relative advantages (ventricular catheter, subdural bolt for small ventricles).

OBJECTIVE 7

Minimum Level of Achievement for Passing

The student should:

A. Provide a differential diagnosis of a delayed rise in ICP that includes reaccumulation of intracerebral hematoma, recurrent subdural hematoma, and cerebral edema.

B. Choose to perform a CT scan and discuss the role of CT in establishing the cause of the increased ICP.

C. Describe the mechanisms and role of body position, respiratory control, fluid management, pain control, and drugs in management of intracranial hypertension.

Honors Level of Achievement

The student should:

A. Provide the doses of mannitol (1 g/kg i.v. single dose or 1/4 g/kg q8h) and furosemide (1 mg/kg single dose, 1/4–1/2 mg/kg q8h) to be administered and the desired level of PCO_2

(25–30 mm Hg) to be achieved when transtentorial herniation threatens to occur.

B. Recognize that marked increase in serum osmolality and hypokalemia restrict the use of mannitol and furosemide, respectively.

OBJECTIVE 8

Minimum Level of Achievement for Passing

The student should:

A. Recognize the presence of a spinal cord lesion and its level and explain how the physical examination leads to those conclusions.

B. Recognize that the cause of the spinal cord lesion is probably unrecognized spinal trauma.

C. Recognize the need to confirm the diagnosis radiologically and to provide external stability to the spine before conducting any studies.

D. Discuss the factors involved in the maintenance of spinal stability (the three-column concept — disruption of two of the three columns causes instability).

Honors Level of Achievement

The student should:

A. Recognize that the spinal lesion is not complete and that incomplete lesions have the potential to recover.

B. Explain the significance of the level of reflex activity, presence of spasticity or flaccidity, and state of motor tone in weakened or paralyzed limbs in lesion localization (complete cord injury is associated with flaccid hypotropic paralysis below the level of the lesion, with loss of deep tendon reflexes and rectal tone).

OBJECTIVE 9

Minimum Level of Achievement for Passing

The student should:

A. Order a CT or MRI scan and describe the relative merits of each as well as the expected findings for each study.

B. Explain the rationale for reduction of cervical spine fracture dislocations.

C. Explain the role of skeletal traction in the closed reduction of cervical spine fracture dislocation.

D. Describe the halo fixation device.

E. Explain the rationale for surgical treatment of cervical spinal cord injuries sustained with fracture dislocation of the cervical spine. Both the role of decompression and of internal fixation and fusion should be addressed.

Honors Level of Achievement

The student should:

A. Recognize that previous craniotomy poses potential problems for the use of halo traction or vest.

B. Explain why operative treatment is better than external fixation alone.

C. Recognize that bone fusion alone is not sufficient, but that internal fixation with metal is required.

OBJECTIVE 10

Minimum Level of Achievement for Passing

The student should:

A. Perform a physical examination and mention both testing the neck for stiffness (realizing this test is limited because of the patient's spinal injury) and any previous neck surgery.

B. Recognize the clinical features of bacterial meningitis from the recent history and physical findings.

C. Proceed with a lumbar puncture after an enhanced CT scan has eliminated possibility of brain abscess or other intracranial mass.

D. Explain the significance of CSF findings in the diagnosis of bacterial meningitis, including the WBC count and differential and the level of CSF glucose.

E. Know the indications for lumbar puncture.

Honors Level of Achievement

The student should:

A. Recognize the relationship between a compound skull fracture extending into the frontal sinus and the development of meningitis.

B. In view of this relationship, elicit a history of clear fluid draining from the patient's nose for the past 2 days.

OBJECTIVE 11

Minimum Level of Achievement for Passing

The student should:

A. Make a diagnosis of CSF rhinorrhea.

B. Recommend and describe the need to test nasal drainage to ascertain that it is CSF. The student should describe how this can be done at the bedside (ring test, glucose strip).

C. Be aware of the role of isotope cisternography or positive contrast CT cisternography in the localization of a CSF fistula.

D. Describe the indications for operative repair of the CFS fistula.

Honors Level of Achievement

The student should recognize that ICP may have become secondarily elevated by hydrocephalus and opened a CSF fistula through the fracture site.

OBJECTIVE 12

Minimum Level of Achievement for Passing

The student should:
  A. Discuss differential diagnosis, recognizing hydrocephalus to be a complication of head trauma and/or meningitis.
  B. Discuss the role of obtaining serum drug levels, performing a lumbar puncture, and doing a CT scan in performing the differential diagnosis.
  C. Recognize the clinical and radiological indications for operative treatment of hydrocephalus.
  D. Offer appropriate operative therapy.

Honors Level of Achievement

The student should list the complications of various operative procedures in the light of the recent abdominal surgery.

Case 2

A 46-year-old right-handed female is sent from her place of work to the emergency room on Friday afternoon with a sudden severe headache that made her pass out. You are called as the consulting neurosurgeon to see her. Vital signs are: temperature, 38.6°C; pulse, 110/minute; BP, 140/96 mm Hg; respiratory rate, 20/minute.

OBJECTIVE 1

The student should elicit the following history and physical examination findings.
  A. Onset and severity of headache (sudden; worst she ever had in her life).
  B. Length of unconsciousness (about 30 seconds).
  C. Vomiting (none).
  D. History of headaches or hypertension (none).
  E. Medications (takes none).
  F. History of easily bruising or bleeding (none).
  G. History of trauma (none).
  H. Alertness (patient is awake and alert; neck slightly stiff).
  I. Photophobia (yes).
  J. Evidence of bruising or ecchymoses (none).

OBJECTIVE 2

The student should make a tentative diagnosis, give a list of other possible diagnoses, and order the appropriate tests to establish the correct diagnosis.

OBJECTIVE 3

The student should pursue further diagnostic tests after CT scan is negative for hematoma, mass lesion, or subarachnoid hemorrhage.

OBJECTIVE 4

Lumbar puncture reveals occiput posterior (OP) 250 mm H_2O, fluid pink (does not clear), red blood cells (RBC) 1500/mm³, WBC 25/mm³, polys 10%, lymphs 25%, total protein 53 g/dL, glucose 70%. The student should provide a differential diagnosis of subarachnoid hemorrhage and order the appropriate tests to differentiate between the possibilities.

OBJECTIVE 5

Arteriogram shows a 10-mm aneurysm at the junction of the left internal carotid artery and the posterior cerebral artery. The student should describe the care of a patient with a subarachnoid hemorrhage while awaiting surgery and recommend when to perform it.

OBJECTIVE 6

The evening following the arteriogram the left pupil becomes dilated and the left eyelid droops. The student should reassess the situation and make recommendations for management.

OBJECTIVE 7

On the fifth day following surgery a nurse calls because of a change in neurologic status. The student should perform a neurologic examination (the patient is drowsy with slurred speech and expressive aphasia, the right hand grasp is slightly weak, the ICP has risen from 8 to 16 mm Hg) and offer a differential diagnosis.

OBJECTIVE 8

The student should order the appropriate tests to establish the diagnosis:
  A. CT scan (normal except for brain swelling the left frontal lobe).
  B. Transcranial Doppler testing (reveals increased velocity in the left middle cerebral artery).
  C. Cerebral arteriography (reveals segmental vasospasm of the left internal carotid artery).

OBJECTIVE 9

The student should order appropriate therapy.

Achievement Level

OBJECTIVE 1

Minimum Level of Achievement for Passing

The student should:
  A. Demonstrate a knowledge of the symptoms of subarachnoid hemorrhage by asking for a history including the items listed under Objective 1, A-G.
  B. Demonstrate knowledge of the signs of subarachnoid hemorrhage, including the items noted under Objective 1, H-J.

Honors Level of Achievement

The student should:
A. Search for symptoms of a recent previous headache that might be indicative of a signal bleed.
B. Search for a family history of subarachnoid hemorrhage, hypertension, or polycystic kidneys.

OBJECTIVE 2

Minimum Level of Achievement for Passing

The student should:
A. List the conditions that mimic subarachnoid hemorrhage (intraparenchymal bleeding, embolic stroke).
B. Explain the limitations of CT scan and MRI scan in the diagnosis of intracranial bleeding (will not demonstrate aneurysms; MRI may not identify subarachnoid hemorrhage).
C. Be able to give two reasons why the CT scan should be ordered before a lumbar puncture is considered.

Honors Level of Achievement

The student should demonstrate knowledge of where to look for subarachnoid blood on the CT scan.

OBJECTIVE 3

Minimum Level of Achievement for Passing

The student should proceed to lumbar puncture and explain the rationale for lumbar puncture in a patient suspected of having a subarachnoid hemorrhage when the CT scan is negative.

Honors Level of Achievement

The student should be able to differentiate between a traumatic lumbar puncture and a subarachnoid hemorrhage.

OBJECTIVE 4

Minimum Level of Achievement for Passing

The student should:
A. Be able to provide a list of possible causes of subarachnoid hemorrhage.
B. Proceed with angiography and discuss its role in establishing the diagnosis of aneurysmal subarachnoid hemorrhage.

Honors Level of Achievement

The student should explain the need to visualize all major cerebral vessels to rule out the presence of multiple aneurysms.

OBJECTIVE 5

Minimum Level of Achievement for Passing

The student should:

A. Demonstrate knowledge that medication to control BP, nimodipine to protect against the effects of vasospasm, analgesia to relieve headache, mild sedation to relieve anxiety, soft foods, and stool softeners are useful in the conservative management of patients with subarachnoid hemorrhage.
B. Know the importance of neurologic status in prognosis.
C. Be aware that early surgery in good grade patients generally is considered indicated and that emergent surgery in moribund patients is indicated only if a scan reveals a significant intraparenchymal hematoma.

Honors Level of Achievement

The student should be aware of the risks of delayed surgery, including rebleeding (greatest in the first 2 days after initial hemorrhage) and vasospasm (more safely treated after the aneurysm has been clipped).

OBJECTIVE 6

Minimum Level of Achievement for Passing

The student should:
A. Explain that aneurysmal enlargement is the cause of the third nerve palsy. The student should state that ptosis with a dilated pupil with or without medial rectus palsy should always raise the suspicion of an enlarging aneurysm even in the absence of a history of subarachnoid hemorrhage.
B. Explain why the above findings are important and what response should be made to this situation.

OBJECTIVE 7

Minimum Level of Achievement for Passing

The student should:
A. Perform a complete neurologic examination.
B. Offer a list of at least three and preferably four causes for the change in neurologic status (rebleed, vasospasm, hydrocephalus, electrolyte imbalance, cerebral edema).

Honors Level of Achievement

The student should be able to discuss the pathogenesis of vasospasm and relate this to its usual time of occurrence.

OBJECTIVE 8

Minimum Level of Achievement for Passing

The student should:
A. Be able to select the appropriate tests and explain the findings that each demonstrates.
B. Arrive at the cause of the patient's deterioration based upon the test results.

Honors Level of Achievement

The student should explain the limitations and potential complications of each test.

OBJECTIVE 9

Minimum Level of Achievement for Passing

The student should be able to explain the principles and methods for treating the problem (hemodilution, volume expansion, hypertension, calcium channel blocker).

Case 3

As the neurosurgeon on call, you are asked to evaluate a 55-year-old female for seizures. When you see her, her vital signs are: temperature, 38.8°C; pulse, 100/minute and regular; respiratory rate, 16/minute; BP, 135/80 mm Hg.

OBJECTIVE 1

The student should elicit the following salient points of history:
  A. The patient has had three seizures in the past 2 months. There is no previous history of seizures.
  B. The seizures are stereotyped. They begin with uncontrollable shaking of the right leg, which progresses to the right arm and face. Witnesses have told her that when she loses consciousness the seizures become generalized.
  C. The patient has noted some numbness of the right leg for about 6 months. It began in the right foot and has slowly progressed to the level of the thigh.
  D. The patient is right handed.
  E. There is no history of weight loss, hemoptysis, or hematuria. She has not had a breast examination for 2 years.

OBJECTIVE 2

The student should demonstrate the following findings on the physical examination.
  A. The patient is awake and alert and oriented to person, place, and time, but her speech is somewhat slow and hesitant.
  B. Although her right leg is strong, she drags it slightly when she walks.
  C. Position sense is decreased in the right great toe.
  D. The fundi are normal. Pupils are equal and small and react.

OBJECTIVE 3

The student should offer a differential diagnosis:
  A. To include brain tumor as well as other disorders.
  B. To differentiate among types of brain tumors.

OBJECTIVE 4

The student should order the appropriate tests to differentiate between these possibilities.
  A. CT or MRI scan (shows a homogeneously enhancing 4-cm round lesion attached to the sagittal sinus posterior to the coronal suture and extending to the left of the midline).
  B. A left internal carotid arteriogram (which shows a vascular 4-cm round lesion that partially occludes the sagittal sinus; a large vein draining the post-Rolandic parietal cortex is posteriorly displaced by the tumor).
  C. A left external carotid arteriogram (shows a significant meningeal artery supplying the tumor).

OBJECTIVE 5

The student should arrive at a specific histologic diagnosis.

OBJECTIVE 6

The student should be able to apprise the patient of some of the operative risks and of the factors related to the prognosis.

Achievement Level
OBJECTIVE 1

Minimum Level of Achievement for Passing

The student should:
  A. Elicit and explore details of the neurologic history and other pertinent historical details.
  B. The student should recognize the significance of a 6-month history of progressive neurologic deficit in the differential diagnosis of the problem.

Honors Level of Achievement

Based upon the progression of the seizure, the patient should be able to localize the mass to the left hemisphere in the region of the Rolandic fissure.

OBJECTIVE 2

Minimum Level of Achievement for Passing

The student should:
  A. Perform a complete neurologic examination.
  B. Based on the physical findings, be able to lateralize the lesion.

C. Based upon the physical findings, localize the lesion more precisely along the medial to lateral as well as the anterior-posterior dimension of the hemisphere.

OBJECTIVE 3

Minimum Level of Achievement for Passing

The student should:
  A. Include brain tumor in the diagnostic possibilities, as well as arteriovenous malformation (AVM), tuberculosis (TB), posttraumatic or postinfectious epilepsy, and brain abscess. The student should also list the common tumors found in the brain.
  B. Demonstrate knowledge of the site of origin of primary intrinsic and extrinsic tumors.

Honors Level of Achievement

The student should:
  A. Demonstrate knowledge of the biologic behavior of these tumors and state which two or three specific types are most likely.
  B. Be able to identify the most common sites of origin of cerebral metastases (lung, breast, kidney, gastrointestinal, skin, thyroid).

OBJECTIVE 4

Minimum Level of Achievement for Passing

The student should:
  A. Demonstrate knowledge of the unenhanced and enhanced CT and MRI findings in each of the tumors under consideration.
  B. Recognize that involvement of the sagittal sinus makes arteriography necessary.

Honors Level of Achievement

The student should:
  A. State that the arteriographic picture of a tumor with blood supply from the external carotid circulation coupled with the CT or MRI findings is most diagnostic of one particular tumor type and why.
  B. Describe the radiologic workup to be undertaken if CT, MRI, or arteriographic findings are not characteristic of meningioma or glioma.

OBJECTIVE 5

Minimum Level of Achievement for Passing

The student should be able diagnose a parasagittal meningioma and state the features characteristic of this condition (history, physical examination, and radiology).

Honors Level of Achievement

The student should be able to differentiate among falcine, parasagittal, and convexity meningiomas.

OBJECTIVE 6

Minimum Level of Achievement for Passing

The student should:
  A. Recognize meningioma as a benign tumor.
  B. Know that the incidence of symptomatic recurrence is directly related to the tumor burden left behind.
  C. Realize that cure is only achieved with total resection of the tumor and its site of dural origin.

Honors Level of Achievement

The student should know that bitemporal hemianopia with loss of smell sense is associated with meningioma of the olfactory nerve.

Case 4

A 50-year-old white male is referred for evaluation of neck and right arm pain.

OBJECTIVE 1

The student should obtain an accurate history, including the pertinent positives and negatives:
  A. The pain began 3 weeks ago without precipitating cause.
  B. It radiates down over the right shoulder along the radial border of the arm into the thumb and second two digits. Pain is also present along the medial border of the scapula.
  C. It is an aching pain exacerbated by coughing, sneezing, or straining.
  D. There is associated numbness in the thumb and second two digits.
  E. The pain does not waken the patient at night.
  F. There is no difficulty with gait and there has been no change in bladder habits.

OBJECTIVE 2

The student should perform a physical examination to elicit the following findings.
  A. There is tenderness over the cervical spine to the right of the midline. Range of motion of the neck is limited by pain, especially of neck flexion and right head tilt.
  B. There is very mild weakness of the right biceps, with a decreased right biceps jerk.
  C. There is mild hypalgesia limited to the thumb and second two digits.
  D. Phalen's sign, Tinel's sign at the wrist, and Adson's sign are absent.
  E. The neurologic examination of the lower extremities is normal. The pupils are equal and reactive to light. There is no ptosis.

OBJECTIVE 3

The student should discuss the differential diagnosis, giving reasons for choosing the most likely diagnostic possibility and for excluding each of the others.

OBJECTIVE 4

The student should make a diagnosis and initiate a management plan.

OBJECTIVE 5

The patient fails to improve and returns 3 weeks later. The physical examination remains unchanged. The student should describe the next steps to be taken.
  A. Cervical spine x-rays (show narrowing of the intervertebral disk space at C-5 to C-6 in the lateral view; oblique views show osteoarthritis with slight encroachment of the neuronal foramen at C-5 to C-6 and C-6 to C-7).
  B. MRI (suggests but only vaguely demonstrates a soft tissue mass in front of the spinal cord to the right of the midline and extending into the neural foramen at C-5 to C-6).

OBJECTIVE 6

The student should ask whether the patient considers the problem severe. If the patient does, the student should ascertain whether there is a surgically correctable lesion by scheduling tests.

OBJECTIVE 7

CT-myelogram demonstrates root sleeve amputation at C-5 to C-6. The student should relate what the patient should be told about possible surgical treatment for the problem.

Achievement Level

OBJECTIVE 1

Minimum Level of Achievement for Passing

The student should:
  A. Be able to obtain a complete history of the condition and elicit pertinent positive and negative events.
  B. The student should realize that the historical data points to compression of the C-6 nerve root.

OBJECTIVE 2

Minimum Level of Achievement for Passing

The student should:
  A. Demonstrate knowledge of the neurologic examination and of which portions are especially relevant tothis patient.
  B. Realize that the physical findings localize the lesion to the C-6 nerve root.

Honors Level of Achievement

The student should be able to tell the difference between C-6 root compression and median nerve compression by physical examination.

OBJECTIVE 3

Minimum Level of Achievement for Passing

The student should:
  A. Offer a differential diagnosis, which includes herniated cervical disk, cervical spondylosis, spinal metastasis, and carpal tunnel syndrome, but not Pancoast tumor or thoracic outlet syndrome and explain why.
  B. Know the presenting symptoms and signs of each of the diagnostic possibilities.

Honors Level of Achievement

The student should be able to identify the specific neural elements that are compressed in a C-6 to C-7 herniated disk, in Pancoast syndrome, in thoracic outlet compression, in a C-5 to C-6 herniated disk, and in carpal tunnel compression.

OBJECTIVE 4

Minimum Level of Achievement for Passing

The student should:
  A. Recognize that the initial treatment of a patient with a cervical strain or with herniated cervical disk and little neurologic deficit is conservative and that radiologic studies are not yet needed.
  B. List factors which would suggest that there is a different diagnosis and which should lead to early radiologic study.
  C. Provide a comprehensive plan of therapy (conservative).

Honors Level of Achievement

The student should state the contraindications (asthma, nasal polyps, peptic ulcer) to use of anti-inflammatory agents and the common complications (headache, gastrointestinal upset and bleeding).

OBJECTIVE 5

Minimum Level of Achievement for Passing

The student should:
  A. Recognize the need for definitive diagnostic tests given the lack of response to conservative therapy.
  B. Understand that the cervical spine x-rays are compatible with discogenic disease and early osteoarthritis in the cervical spine but that these are not diagnostic of the problem.
  C. Be able to describe the findings expected on CT or MRI scan in a patient with a herniated disk, spinal metastasis, spinal stenosis from osteoarthritis, or carpal tunnel syndrome.

Honors Level of Achievement

The student should:
A. Be able to describe the pertinent x-ray findings, if any, in each of the differential diagnostic choices (Objective 3, Achievement Level A).
B. Be able to describe the pertinent CT and MRI findings, if any, in each of these differential diagnostic choices.
C. Be able to describe the value of electrical studies of muscle and nerve in establishing a differential diagnosis.

OBJECTIVE 6

Minimum Level of Achievement for Passing

The student should suggest that a CT-myelogram be done, explain the rationale for the use of CT myelography in the diagnosis of disk disease, and note the importance of MRI as a frequent first choice in pursuing this diagnosis.

Honors Level of Achievement

The student should describe the finding expected on CT myelography in a patient with a herniated disk at the expected level.

OBJECTIVE 7

Minimum Level of Achievement for Passing

The student should:
A. Explain the nature of the condition.
B. Explain the object of the operation.
C. Be able to explain the likelihood that pain will be relieved and the likelihood of recurrence.
D. Understand that the objective of surgery is the relief of root compression and radicular pain.

Honors Level of Achievement

The student should:
A. Explain the possible major complications of the anterior and posterior approach for cervical disk disease.
B. Know that the incidence of failure to relieve limb pain is 5–10%, the likelihood of late recurrence at the same level is 5%, and the incidence of occurrence at the adjacent level is 5%.

Case 5

You are called by the neonatal unit to see a newborn male with a myelomeningocele.

OBJECTIVE 1

The student should elicit the pertinent historical facts:
A. Date and time of birth.
B. Duration and nature of pregnancy.
C. Type of delivery.
D. Family history of spina bifida.
E. Any information gleaned from prenatal ultrasound studies.

OBJECTIVE 2

The student should obtain the following physical findings:
A. Size and location (6-cm myelomeningocele extending from T-12 to L-4).
B. Whether there is any leaking (the myelomeningocele is open and leaking spinal fluid).
C. Lower extremity motor function (trace flexion at the hips and no motion below).
D. Anal reflex testing (no anal wink).
E. Lower extremity sensory function (there is an apparent sensory level at the groin).
F. Head circumference (34.0 cm).
G. Status of anterior fontanelle (full but not tense).

OBJECTIVE 3

The student should order the appropriate studies, including:
A. Spine x-rays (demonstrate a mild kyphosis).
B. Ultrasound of the head (demonstrates mild hydrocephalus) and of abdomen (normal kidneys).

OBJECTIVE 4

The student should plan appropriate therapy.

OBJECTIVE 5

Surgery demonstrates a large myelomeningocele containing both neural placode and nerve roots. The student should plan appropriate follow-up of the neurologic condition in the postoperative period.

OBJECTIVE 6

Wound healing proceeds without incident, leg motion and anal wink are unchanged, and head growth is progressive, reaching 35.5 cm 1 week after surgery. The student should choose a next step in patient care:
A. Repeat ultrasound (demonstrates progressive ventricular dilation).
B. Make a diagnosis and formulate a plan of treatment.

OBJECTIVE 7

The patient is seen in follow-up clinic 2 months after discharge. His mother states he has been fussy and lethargic for the past week. The student should

perform a physical examination, including inspection of:
  A. The myelomeningocele repair site (bulging).
  B. The fontanelle (full and pulsatile).
  C. The head circumference (37.0 cm).
  D. Upward gaze (impaired).
  E. The shunt (collapses when pressed upon and does not fill).

OBJECTIVE 8

The student should offer a diagnosis and order the appropriate tests.

OBJECTIVE 9

The scan reveals the ventricles to be dilated and the shunt is revised. Following the revision, the patient does well and is discharged. Two weeks later, the child reappears with a temperature of 38.2°C. He is irritable and fussy. The fontanelle is scaphoid. Upward gaze is normal. The shunt pumps and fills well. The student should offer a diagnosis (including the need to rule out shunt infection) and should arrange for appropriate tests.
  A. CT scan (demonstrates decrease in ventricular size).
  B. Shunt tap (demonstrates an opening pressure of 50 mm H_2O. The fluid is slightly turbid. Cells $150/mm^3$, polys 100%, lymphs 50%; glucose, 35 mg/dL; protein, 105 mg/dL).

OBJECTIVE 10

The student should offer a treatment plan.

Achievement Level

OBJECTIVE 1

Minimum Level of Achievement for Passing

The student should be able to obtain a pertinent history.

Honors Level of Achievement

The student should:
  A. State the role of γ-fetoprotein and ultrasound in the management of myelomeningocele.
  B. Be aware of the possible role of premature rupture of the membranes in the contamination of an open myelomeningocele.

OBJECTIVE 2

Minimum Level of Achievement for Passing

The student should perform a pertinent physical examination.

Honors Level of Achievement

The student should note the presence of other serious congenital defects (hydrocephalus, hip dislocation, bladder dysfunction, scoliosis).

OBJECTIVE 3

Minimum Level of Achievement for Passing

The student should identify the appropriate studies and state their expected findings.

Honors Level of Achievement

The student should:
  A. Be able to relate the association of hydrocephalus to the level of the myelomeningocele.
  B. Name two possible mechanisms for development of hydrocephalus in patients with myelomeningocele (Chiari II deformity, meningitis).
  C. Order an abdominal ultrasound to check the configuration of the kidneys.

OBJECTIVE 4

Minimum Level of Achievement for Passing

The student should:
  A. Be able to give the rationale for surgical repair and closure of the myelomeningocele.
  B. Be able to give the principles and steps of the operative repair.

Honors Level of Achievement

The student should evaluate early versus delayed closure of the defect and explain the possible complications of each.

OBJECTIVE 5

Minimum Level of Achievement for Passing

The student should list three or four common postoperative problems (hydrocephalus, leg dysfunction, scoliosis, meningitis).

OBJECTIVE 6

Minimum Level of Achievement for Passing

The student should:
  A. Explain the mechanisms that cause hydrocephalus in children with myelomeningocele.
  B. Explain the principles of a ventricular shunting procedure.
  C. List the complications of the different shunt procedures.

Honors Level of Achievement

The student should be aware that a collapsed shunt may be found in slit-like ventricles because of an overfunctioning shunt or because of an obstructed ventricular catheter.

OBJECTIVE 8

Minimum Level of Achievement for Passing

The student should:

A. Make a preliminary diagnosis of shunt malfunction.
B. Explain the information to be gained from plain x-rays of the head, neck, chest, and abdomen.
C. Be able to describe the CT or MRI findings in hydrocephalus and what to do if it is found.

Honors Level of Achievement

The student should be able to explain the role of shunt tap in the diagnosis of shunt malfunction and know the normal ventricular pressure in a neonate (<80 mm H_2O).

OBJECTIVE 9

Minimum Level of Achievement for Passing

The student should:
A. Consider shunt infection as a strong diagnostic possibility.
B. Order a CT scan, perform a shunt tap, and describe the findings expected on the basis of the working diagnosis.
C. Be aware that the demonstration of bacteria in the ventricular fluid (or in the blood of a patient with a ventriculoatrial shunt) is necessary to make a diagnosis of shunt infection.
D. State the most common infecting organism (*Staphylococcus epidermidis*).

Honors Level of Achievement

The student should be aware that the greatest risk factor for shunt infection is recent shunt placement.

OBJECTIVE 10

Minimum Level of Achievement

The student should describe the treatment of shunt infection.

Case 6

A 34-year-old female presents with a complaint of difficulty walking.

OBJECTIVE 1

The student should elicit the following pertinent history.
A. The patient developed pain between her shoulders about 6 months ago.
B. The pain began to radiate around the left side of the chest 1 month ago.
C. The patient began to have difficulty walking 2 weeks ago.
D. Sphincter function is normal.

E. One week ago, she noted swelling and a bruise about her left ankle but no pain.
F. The patient is not a drug abuser; has had no recent surgery in the area of pain; has no history of fever, chills, or malaise.
G. The student should offer an initial differential diagnosis.

OBJECTIVE 2

The student should elicit the following physical findings.
A. Tenderness at the level of the T-7 spine.
B. 4/5 strength in the right leg with hyperreflexia and a Babinski sign. Reflexes in the other three extremities are normal.
C. Decreased vibratory and position sense in the right leg.
D. Decreased pin sensation from the left upper quadrant on down, including the entire left lower extremity.
E. Rectal examination (demonstrates normal tone).
F. Fever (none).
G. Breast lumps, hepatosplenomegaly or adenopathy (none).

OBJECTIVE 3

The student should offer a differential diagnosis.

OBJECTIVE 4

The student should order the appropriate tests and x-ray examinations to localize the lesion and arrive at a diagnosis.
A. Chest film (normal).
B. Anteroposterior (AP) and lateral thoracic spine films (normal).
C. MRI scan with enhancement (demonstrates an enhancing lesion anterior to the spinal cord in the right anterolateral quadrant of the canal).
D. The student should give a differential diagnosis.

OBJECTIVE 5

The student should be able to describe the operative approach and the operative findings.

OBJECTIVE 6

Assume that the student has elicited the same history as in Objective 1, except that the duration of pain is only 2 weeks and that the duration of difficulty with sensation and walking is only 1 day. Assume that examination reveals bilateral sensory and motor loss in all modalities, which is almost total below T-7; that reflexes are 2+ in the upper and 3+ in the lower extremities with bilateral

Babinski's signs. The student should offer a tentative diagnosis and some sense of its urgency.

OBJECTIVE 7

The student should order appropriate tests.
A. Thoracic spine film (shows loss of pedicle at T-10 on left).
B. MRI scan (shows lucent areas in marrow of T-3, T-7, and T-10 vertebral bodies with evidence of a soft tissue mass behind the vertebral body of T-7 displacing the spinal cord posteriorly as a thin ribbon).

OBJECTIVE 8

The student should outline the factors that determine a management plan.

OBJECTIVE 9

The student should describe postoperative care.

Achievement Level

OBJECTIVE 1

Minimum Level of Achievement for Passing

The student should:
A. Be able to elicit the pertinent historical findings.
B. Indicate what processes are the likely causes of these symptoms, including spinal tumor, abscess, osteomyelitis, and disk herniation. The student should rank such entities as multiple sclerosis, Guillain-Barre, diabetic neuropathy, or syrinx as unlikely and explain why.

Honors Level of Achievement

The student should know the history typical of intramedullary, intradural extramedullary, and extradural tumors, including peak age of onset, types of pain, as well as usual duration of pain and other neurologic symptoms before diagnosis.

OBJECTIVE 2

Minimum Level of Achievement for Passing

The student should:
A. Be able to perform a pertinent physical examination.
B. Recognize the presence of a Brown-Sequard syndrome and describe it as a hemicord syndrome.

Honors Level of Achievement

The student should:
A. Identify the clinical hallmarks observed on physical examination in cases of intramedullary tumor, intradural extramedullary tumor, and extradural tumor.
B. Recognize that the most common cause of Brown-Sequard syndrome is a spinal tumor.

C. Be able to identify at least two types of intramedullary tumor, two types of intradural extramedullary tumors, and the most common type of extradural tumor.
D. Be able to explain why a Brown-Sequard syndrome is commonly found with extramedullary tumors but not with intramedullary ones.

OBJECTIVE 3

Minimum Level of Achievement for Passing

The student should focus upon a diagnosis of tumor or abscess, but some other conditions such as syrinx, thoracic disk, and discitis should be considered and tentatively rejected.

OBJECTIVE 4

Minimum Level of Achievement for Passing

The student should:
A. Order the appropriate tests.
B. Describe the plain x-ray findings, characteristics of intramedullary extradural tumors, and extradural tumors.
C. Arrive at a presumptive diagnosis of extramedullary intradural tumor and offer possible histologies.

Honors Level of Achievement

The student should:
A. Explain which specific histology would be favored.
B. Describe the MRI findings with intramedullary tumors and with extramedullary tumors.

OBJECTIVE 5

Minimum Level of Achievement for Passing

The student should:
A. Know the anatomy of the vertebral column, including the vertebral bodies, the intervertebral disks, the pedicles, the facets, the lamina, and the spines.
B. Identify the osseous structures that will be removed in the posterior approach to the tumor.
C. Realize that the dura must be opened to see the tumor and remove it.

Honors Level of Achievement

The student should:
A. Understand that spinal cord function can be monitored during surgery and be able to explain which tracts are being tested when somatosensory-evoked responses are measured.
B. State the limitations of retraction in attempts to remove a tumor beneath the cord and should

propose an appropriate means of extracting such a tumor when exposure from retraction is limited.

OBJECTIVE 6

Minimum Level of Achievement for Passing

The student should:
A. Recognize that the most important diagnostic possibility is tumor or abscess and that metastatic tumor is the most probable specific diagnosis.
B. Recognize that the development of profound weakness and sensory loss within a period of a day or two requires emergent diagnosis and treatment.

OBJECTIVE 7

Minimum Level of Achievement for Passing

The student should:
A. Order the appropriate tests.
B. Recognize that x-ray changes at T-10 do not explain a sensory loss extending up to T-7.
C. Recognize that T-10 changes are consistent with metastatic disease and that this is the likely diagnosis.
D. Order an MRI because there is a need to look for other lesions, especially lesions at T-7 or higher.

Honors Level of Achievement

The student should:
A. Recognize that the lesion responsible for the patient's deficits may lie at a level higher than T-7.
B. Know which metastatic lesions cause osteoblastic lesions (prostate, lymphoma, thyroid, breast), while recognizing that some of these (all but the first) may cause only osteolytic lesions.

C. Recognize that most metastatic lesions of the spine are osteolytic.
D. Know the x-ray and MRI findings of vertebral osteomyelitis and stress the destruction of the intervertebral disk in osteomyelitis compared with its preservation in cases of spinal metastases.

OBJECTIVE 8

Minimum Level of Achievement for Passing

The student should:
A. Recognize that rapid treatment is mandatory.
B. Recognize the difference in therapy for very radiosensitive lesions and those of unknown or lesser radiosensitivity.

Honors Level of Achievement

The student should:
A. Recognize which approaches are suitable and why, if surgery is to be done.
B. Understand that the operation may also require internal fixation and fusion.

OBJECTIVE 9

Minimum Level of Achievement for Passing

The student's postoperative plans should include bladder catheterization or careful monitoring of the need for catheterization; good pulmonary toilet; placement of patient on special bedding or rotating bed to avoid pressure sores; delay in instituting feeding; postoperative steroids; monitoring of vital signs and blood gases.

Honors Level of Achievement

The student should recognize that long-term management should include passive exercises, a bowel regimen, monitoring for autonomic hyperreflexia, metastatic survey, physical rehabilitation program, radiation therapy, and oncology consultation.

9

Urology: Diseases of the Genitourinary System

Case 1

You are a urology resident in the clinic when a 55-year-old male presents for an annual physical examination that is unremarkable except for an enlarged left side of the prostate. The patient has had voiding dysfunction and nocturia six times during the last 2 months.

OBJECTIVE 1

The student should outline the initial evaluation.
  A. Uroflow pattern.
  B. Rectal examination.
  C. Other pertinent laboratory studies (acid phosphatase, prostatic specific antigen [PSA], urine culture, urinalysis).
  D. Postvoid residual urine.

OBJECTIVE 2

The student should begin a diagnostic evaluation, including a digital rectal examination.
  A. Digital rectal examination reveals an indurated left side of the prostate with an absence of the prostate seminal vesical junction. The patient also has some enlarge-ment of the bladder with a palpable bladder midway up to the umbilicus.
  B. A transrectal or transperineal biopsy of the prostate is done.
  C. If the biopsy is positive, the patient workup should include: PSA, acid phosphatase, a bone scan, and a pelvic computed tomography [CT] scan.
  D. The pelvic CT scan reveals iliac lymphad-enopathy; the bone scan demonstrates disease in the axial skeleton.
  E. The patient is diagnosed as having metastatic carcinoma.

OBJECTIVE 3

The student should be able to describe appropriate surgical intervention and treatment.

  A. Bilateral orchiectomy.
  B. Luteinizing hormone releasing hormone [LHRH] agonists, adrenal blockers, and anti-androgen therapy.
  C. Consider option of no treatment if asymptomatic.

Achievement Level

OBJECTIVE 1

Minimum Level of Achievement for Passing

The student should:
  A. Ask for a basic history and appropriate laboratory tests.
  B. Discuss possible diagnosis of enlarged prostate and voiding dysfunction.

Honors Level of Achievement

The student should discuss an appropriate workup for a patient with a prostatic mass and with voiding symptoms of relatively short duration. Tests should include PSA, acid phosphatase, bone scan, and CT scan for staging the disease. The tumor's Gleason score should be noted.

OBJECTIVE 2

Minimum Level of Achievement for Passing

The student should:
  A. Consider appropriate diagnostic workup including staging tests and a CT scan.
  B. Understand the need for tissue diagnosis and a biopsy, either transcutaneously or with dissection of the enlarged pelvic lymph nodes.

Honors Level of Achievement

The student should:
  A. Ask for lymph node biopsy and evaluate the bone scan.
  B. Understand that the findings mean disseminated disease and that the patient probably requires therapy.

OBJECTIVE 3

Minimum Level of Achievement for Passing

The student should:
  A. Understand the therapy that should be considered for a patient with metastatic disease.
  B. Understand that most prostate cancers are hormonally mediated.

Honors Level of Achievement

The student should:
  A. Be able to discuss the problem of testosterone flare of unopposed early action of LHRH agonists.
  B. Discuss the side effects of many antiandrogen therapies and how these may influence the patient's response to the disease.
  C. Discuss how acid phosphatase or PSA levels could be used to follow patients who are treated appropriately.

Case 2

You are a family physician and a 53-year-old female presents to you complaining of mild discomfort in her right side, dark urine, and some mild burning on urination for 3 weeks. She states she has had a low-grade temperature for the past several days. Her physical examination reveals mild right flank tenderness, but nothing else of note.

OBJECTIVE 1

The student should outline the initial evaluation of this patient.
  A. History (no history of trauma, exposure to infection, dyspareunia).
  B. Physical examination (palpable mass in the right upper quadrant [RUQ], mildly tender costovertebral angle [CVA], normal pelvic examination).
  C. Complete blood count (CBC — white blood cells [WBC], 6200/mm^3; hematocrit [Hct], 47%; hemoglobin [Hgb], 14.3 g/dL).
  D. Urinalysis (positive for blood, Hgb, negative for other elements).
  E. Other assays (serum lactase dehydrogenase [LDH], 260; other liver enzymes normal, blood urea nitrogen [BUN], 20 mg/dL; creatinine, 1.9).

OBJECTIVE 2

The student should begin a diagnostic evaluation, especially a radiographic one.
  A. Intravenous urography (IVU — small left-sided lower pole calyceal stone measuring approximately 6 mm x 4 mm, nonobstructing; distorted right upper pole collecting system with the kidney being displaced inferiorly and upper pole displaced laterally).
  B. Renal ultrasound (left-sided stone confirmed in lower pole, large solid mass seen in right kidney with no hydronephrosis appreciated).
  C. Abdominal CT scan (large 12-cm mass in upper pole of the right kidney with inferior displacement, no apparent retroperitoneal adenopathy, large right renal vein with medially displaced inferior vena cava, mass enhances with i.v. contrast).
  D. Inferior vena cavagram (tumor thrombus into the right renal vein, extending into the vena cava for about 2 cm and ending below the hepatic veins).
  E. Arteriogram (hypervascular mass about 12 cm in the right kidney with venous "lakes" and pooling of contrast material, neovascularization, single renal artery seen on the right).
  F. Chest x-ray (mild interstitial changes, no masses).
  G. Cystoscopy (mild trigonitis).

OBJECTIVE 3

The student should be able to describe the appropriate surgical intervention for this patient and the appropriate staging.
  A. Radical nephrectomy.
  B. Vena cavotomy with thrombus excision.
  C. Staging (stage TNM T3cNxMO thus far).

Achievement Level

OBJECTIVE 1

Minimum Level of Achievement for Passing

The student should:
  A. Request basic history, physical examination, and laboratory tests, including renal function tests and urinalysis.
  B. Be able to discuss the possible causes of hematuria (i.e., make a differential diagnosis).

Honors Level of Achievement

The student should discuss appropriate workup for hematuria of any type and name its urologic causes.

OBJECTIVE 2

Minimum Level of Achievement for Passing

The student should:
  A. Order at least two of the radiographic tests found in the list and give a rationale for ordering each.
  B. Proceed in a logical fashion through the workup.

Honors Level of Achievement

The student should:
  A. Order the inferior vena cavagram and discuss why it is important.
  B. Include cystoscopy in a hematuria workup.

OBJECTIVE 3

Minimum Level of Achievement for Passing

The student should:
  A. Select the correct surgical procedure.
  B. Be able to stage the tumor.

Honors Level of Achievement

The student should, in addition to discussing the treatment of renal cell cancer:
  A. Be able to differentiate treatment options between superficial and muscle-invading bladder tumors.
  B. Understand that because bladder tumors have a high recurrence rate, intravesical chemotherapy may be necessary.

Case 3

You are a family practitioner when one of your patients, a 60-year-old female, mother of four children, develops incontinence.

OBJECTIVE 1

The student should obtain a thorough history and review of systems, including pertinent negative items.
  A. Urinary leakage (precipitated by coughing, sneezing, hiccups, and lifting heavy objects).
  B. Amount of leakage (patient wears adult protection pads to prevent staining and wetting clothes; changes them three to five times a day; pads are usually quite soaked).
  C. Leakage without straining (none).
  D. Associated urgency with incontinence (none).
  E. Nocturnal enuresis (none).
  F. Diabetes (no).
  G. Urinary tract infections (rarely).
  H. Back injury or surgery (none).
  I. Neurologic deficits (none).
  J. Previous pelvic or abdominal surgery (none).

OBJECTIVE 2

The student should be able to outline a physical examination, laboratory studies, and urodynamic evaluation appropriate to the problem; request findings pertinent to the problem; and interpret the results. The student should diagnose stress incontinence.
  A. Physical findings

  1. Abdominal examination (no surgical scars, nontender abdomen, no masses).
  2. Back (no surgical scars).
  3. Lower extremities (normal motor and sensory function, normal deep tendon reflexes, no Babinski reflex).
  4. Pelvic examination (to be done in lithotomy position with a full bladder).
      a. Introitus (evidence of previous vaginal deliveries).
      b. Perineal sensation and anal sphincter tone (normal).
      c. Cough (reveals rotational descent of bladder neck and urethra, a mild cystocele, and urinary leakage).
  5. Bonney test (after demonstration of leakage: further leakage with coughing is prevented by correcting the descensus with two fingers lateral to the bladder neck; care is taken not to physically occlude the urethra).
  B. Laboratory studies
  1. Urinalysis (normal).
  2. Urine culture (no growth).
  3. Urine cytologies (benign).
  4. Serum chemistries (normal BUN, creatinine, and glucose).
  C. Urodynamic evaluation
  1. Postvoid residual (10 mL).
  2. Cystometrogram (normal compliance, no uninhibited contractions).
  3. Flow rate, electromyograph (EMG), and urethral pressure profile (normal).
  4. Fluoroscopic cystography (mild cystocele with rotational descent of the bladder neck and urethra).

OBJECTIVE 3

The student should explain the basic anatomic concepts involved in the surgical correction of stress urinary incontinence and list and describe the possible procedures for correction.
  A. True stress incontinence occurs as intraabdominal pressure exceeds urethral resting pressure. Normally resting urethral pressure is higher than intravesical pressure due to the urethra's relatively fixed position in the retropubic space. Hypermobility of the urethra due to aging, childbirth, or other causes allows transmission of intravesical or intraabdominal pressure directly to the urethral sphincter, overcoming its normal resting pressure. Urinary incontinence results. A cystocele is not always related to or indicative of stress urinary incontinence.
  B. Elevation of the bladder neck and/or urethra will correct stress urinary incontinence in 90% of cases over 5 years. Two surgical approaches are used. The Marshall-Marchetti-Krantz procedure has been the gold standard of

bladder suspensions. Variants of this procedure are performed through a low, suprapubic incision. The bladder neck is sutured to the pubis to reposition the urethra in its normal location. In another procedure, an easier and faster way to correct stress urinary incontinence, a vaginal approach is used to attach the bladder neck and urethra to the rectus fascia by means of suspension sutures. An artificial sphincter or sling procedure is reserved for severe incontinence resulting from a nonfunctioning urethra.

Achievement Level

OBJECTIVE 1

Minimum Level of Achievement for Passing

The student should:
A. Ask appropriate questions to establish the presence of stress incontinence.
B. Ask the patient to quantitate the amount of leakage.

Honors Level of Achievement

The student should obtain a pertinent negative history of no urge incontinence, nocturnal enuresis, infections, diabetes, back, or pelvic surgery.

OBJECTIVE 2

Minimum Level of Achievement for Passing

The student should:
A. Request findings of a pelvic examination.
B. Request findings of a neurologic examination.
C. Request results of a urinalysis and urine culture.
D. Request results of a cystometrogram.

Honors Level of Achievement

The student should:
A. Request results of complete abdominal, back, pelvic, and lower extremity examinations.
B. Request results of a Bonney test.
C. Request the result of urine cytology and serum chemistries.
D. Request the results of a postvoid residual and cystometrogram (CMG).
E. Diagnose stress urinary incontinence.

OBJECTIVE 3

Minimum Level of Achievement

The student should:
A. Know that the cause of stress incontinence is the descent of the bladder from its proper anatomic position.
B. List the Marshall-Marchetti-Krantz procedure and the Stamey and Raz bladder suspensions as treatment options.

Honors Level of Achievement

The student should:
A. Explain that the rotational descent of the bladder prevents the transmission of intraabdominal pressure to the sphincter and bladder neck and overpowers intrinsic sphincter resistance; explain that surgery should correct the anatomic position of the bladder.
B. Describe the Marshall-Marchetti-Krantz procedure.
C. Describe the Stamey and Raz procedures.

Case 4

A 13-year-old white male presents with acute onset of left testicular pain.

OBJECTIVE 1

The student should establish a differential diagnosis based on physical examination.
A. Obtain a proper history (previous episodes of testicular pain, history of vigorous activity).
B. Perform a complete physical examination (hard, enlarged, tender mass that does not transilluminate, no "blue dot" sign).
C. Establish whether the testicle is palpable and in the normal position (lying high in the scrotum).
D. Perform a differential diagnosis (incarcerated hernia, torsion of testicular appendage, trauma, viral orchitis, epididymoorchitis).
E. Obtain laboratory tests, CBC, urinalysis (no pyuria).

OBJECTIVE 2

The student should outline treatment.
A. Manual detorsion/orchidopexy.
B. Bed rest, antibiotics, and analgesics (not indicated).
C. Observation (not indicated).

OBJECTIVE 3

The student should be aware of the natural history of the disease.
A. Age group usually associated with torsion (teenagers and neonates).
B. Viability of testicle is suspect after 6 hours of torsion.

Achievement Level

OBJECTIVE 1

Minimum Level of Achievement for Passing

The student should recognize that torsion is the most likely diagnosis, that manual detorsion and urgent orchidopexy are the treatments of choice, and that viability and fertility are diminished after 6 hours.

Honors Level of Achievement

The student should discuss an alternate diagnosis of trauma or epididymorchitis based upon a complete physical examination and history taking (pyuria rules out epididymoorchitis).

Case 5

A 6-year-old male with a nonpalpable left testicle is brought into your office by his mother.

OBJECTIVE 1

The student should establish the differential diagnosis based on physical examination.
  A. Conduct physical examination (normal right testicle, normal male genitalia).
  B. Describe possibilities of inguinal testicle versus retractile testicle versus nonpalpable testicle (retractile testis is easily pulled into scrotum).

OBJECTIVE 2

The student should outline treatment.
  A. If retractable testicle, no treatment (will descend at puberty).
  B. If nonpalpable testicle, ultrasound or CT scan and exploration indicated.
  C. Orchidopexy for palpable testicle.

OBJECTIVE 3

The student should be aware of the natural history of the condition.
  A. Know that undescended testicle is associated with fertility aberration as well as increased malignancy.
  B. Know that orchidopexy does not protect the patient from malignancy or future infertility.
  C. Discuss the embryologic etiology of non-descent.

Achievement Level

Minimum Level of Achievement for Passing

The student should demonstrate a knowledge of the three clinical entities associated with an absent testicle and the appropriate treatments for each (anorchia, nondescent, retractile testis).

Honors Level of Achievement

The student should discuss the ramifications of performing or not performing orchidopexy (does not decrease risk of malignancy but allows for earlier diagnosis of malignancy).

Case 6

A 19-year-old white male is found to have a 2-cm mass in the midpole of his right testicle.

OBJECTIVE 1

The student should establish the diagnosis of testicular cancer.
  A. Complete the history and physical examination (how long mass has been present; whether increasing in size or painful; position; whether mass transilluminates; history of infection, trauma, or surgery).
  B. Order testicular ultrasound.
  C. Obtain tumor markers (γ-fetoprotein [AFP], beta-human chorionic gonadotropin (BHCG), LKH, carcinoembryonic antigen [CEA], HCS).

OBJECTIVE 2

The student should outline treatment.
  A. Advise inguinal exploration with orchi-ectomy.
  B. Establish proper staging evaluation with CT scan, chest x-ray, and preoperative and post-operative markers.
  C. Discuss radiation therapy for seminomas and chemotherapeutic regimens for nonseminomas.

Achievement Level

Minimum Level of Achievement for Passing

The student should:
  A. Obtain preoperative markers and discuss an inguinal approach rather than a transscrotal one for an orchiectomy.
  B. Adequately describe the proper staging techniques and distinguish seminomas from nonseminomas.

Honors Level of Achievement

The student should:
  A. Be able to discuss the proper staging of germ cell tumors of the testicle and describe the chemotherapeutic agents involved in therapy of nonseminomatous germ cell tumors.
  B. Be able to contrast radiation therapy to chemotherapeutic regimens.

Case 7

A 26-year-old white male states that he is unable to impregnate his wife despite 2 years of unprotected intercourse.

OBJECTIVE 1

The student should establish a diagnosis.

A. Elicit a complete sexual history including frequency and time of intercourse, childhood illnesses, surgical procedures, problems with puberty, recent viral illnesses, medications or spermicidals, cigarette or marijuana smoking.

B. Perform a complete physical examination with attention to testicular size, consistency, presence of peritesticular organs, visual fields, breasts, escutcheon, position and size of urethral meatus.

C. Obtain serum hormones (testosterone, follicle-stimulating hormone [FSH], luteinizing hormone [LH]).

D. Obtain a semen analysis (postcoital cervical mucus penetration assay, antisperm antibody test, semen fructose level).

OBJECTIVE 2

The student should outline treatment.

A. Describe the role of varicocelectomy and expected outcomes (improved semen in 64% of men leading to pregnancy rate of 35%).

B. Elicit empiric therapy for male factor.

C. Discuss the various drugs and medications that may affect male factor fertility (cimetidine, Macrodantin, Azulfidine decrease fertility).

Achievement Level

Minimum Level of Achievement for Passing

The student should:

A. Demonstrate an ability to obtain a complete history including previous surgical, medical, or anatomical abnormalities that may lead to infertility.

B. Discuss an "adequate" semen analysis (volume 1.5–5.0 mL, density >20 million/mL, motility >60%, grade of motility >2, morphology >60% normal).

Honors Level of Achievement

The student should mention antisperm antibodies and postcoital examination.

Case 8

A 60-year-old white male states that he has been unable to attain erections for the last 2 years.

OBJECTIVE 1

The student should make an evaluation.

A. Obtain a complete history and physical examination.

B. Define the four types of erectile dysfunction (endocrinologic, psychogenic, neurogenic, vasculogenic).

C. Discuss tests in evaluating vasculogenic erectile dysfunction (plethysmography, duplex ultrasound, pharmacocavernosometry).

OBJECTIVE 3

The student should outline treatment.

A. Discuss possible hormonal therapy.

B. Describe the indication and treatment options available for intracavernosal pharmacotherapy.

Achievement Level

Minimum Level of Achievement for Passing

The student should obtain a complete physical examination and history and be able to describe the workup for the four different types of erectile dysfunction.

Honors Level of Achievement

The student should discuss the mechanism of vasculogenic impotence and the problems associated with nocturnal penile tumescence testing.

Case 9

A 19-year-old male involved in a motor vehicle accident has been evaluated by the trauma surgery service and found to be in stable condition. Abdominal radiographs demonstrate multiple pelvic fractures; blood has been noted at the urethral meatus. You have been asked to evaluate the patient for possible urologic trauma.

OBJECTIVE 1

The student should recognize this patient is at high risk for posterior urethral injury because of the presence of a pelvic fracture and blood at the urethral meatus.

OBJECTIVE 2

The student should obtain a pertinent history:

A. A normal urologic and voiding history prior to the motor vehicle accident.

B. Inability to void since the traumatic event.

OBJECTIVE 3

The student should elicit pertinent physical findings:

A. The presence of a scrotal and perineal butterfly hematoma that extends up the abdominal wall under Scarpa's fascia.

B. Rectal examination demonstrating a superiorly displaced prostate gland suggesting a pelvic hematoma.

OBJECTIVE 4

The student should ask for appropriate radiographic studies:
  A. An intravenous pyelogram (IVP) should be performed prior to retrograde ureterography and cystography so that contrast extravasation from the later two studies does not obscure the intravenous pyelogram findings. The IVP demonstrates bilateral normal kidneys and ureters.
  B. Retrograde ureterography demonstrates massive retroperitoneal extravasation of contrast without passage of contrast into the bladder.

OBJECTIVE 5

The student should make the diagnosis of complete disruption of the posterior urethra.

OBJECTIVE 6

The student should discuss the surgical management of this patient.
  A. Immediate repair (cystostomy, evacuate hematoma and bony fragments, repair bladder lacerations, realign urethra by passage of urethral catheter).
  B. Delayed repair (suprapubic cystostomy without urethral realignment; definitive urethroplasty to be performed 3–6 months later if necessary).

OBJECTIVE 7

The student should recognize that although delayed repair inevitably results in urethral stricture, incontinence and impotency rates are far lower in these patients than in patients treated by immediate repair.

Achievement Level

Minimum Level of Achievement for Passing

The student should be able to obtain the relevant history, elicit pertinent physical findings, order appropriate radiographic tests, and make the diagnosis of a urethral laceration.

Honors Level of Achievement

The student should:
  A. Order the radiographic tests in the proper sequence, make the diagnosis of complete posterior urethral rupture, and discuss the management of the patient.
  B. Be able to recognize the advantages and disadvantages of immediate urethral repair versus suprapubic cystostomy and delayed urethral repair.

Case 10

A 67-year-old male complains of a penile mass.

OBJECTIVE 1

The student should obtain the pertinent history.
  A. The penile mass has enlarged slowly over the past 6 months.
  B. The patient is uncircumcised with a phimotic prepuce.
  C. The penile lesion cannot be seen but can be felt through the prepuce.
  D. A foul-smelling purulent drainage is coming from the prepucial sac.

OBJECTIVE 2

The student should elicit pertinent physical findings.
  A. Phimotic prepuce that cannot be retracted.
  B. Foul-smelling purulent drainage from the prepucial sac.
  C. A penile mass, approximately 1.5-cm, which on palpation appears to be localized to the penile glands.
  D. Bilateral inguinal adenopathy present.
  E. No other physical findings of metastatic disease.

OBJECTIVE 3

In the differential diagnosis, the student should strongly consider squamous cell carcinoma of the penis.

OBJECTIVE 4

The student should outline treatment options of the primary lesion.
  A. Penectomy. The student should know that the optimal treatment is partial penectomy if the following criteria are met: the patient has a distal tumor 2 cm or less in size that can be excised with a 2-cm margin of normal tissue, such that the remaining penis is long enough to permit voiding in the standing position. If these criteria cannot be met, then total penectomy and perineal urethrostomy is indicated.
  B. Radiotherapy. The patient should know that the advantage of radiotherapy is penile preservation, but local control is less than that obtained by penectomy.

OBJECTIVE 5

The student should proceed with the clinical staging of the patient.

A. Serum liver function tests (within normal limits).
B. Chest radiograph (no metastatic disease).
C. Bone scan (no metastatic disease).
D. CT of abdomen and pelvis — should be delayed until patient has received 4–6 weeks of antimicrobials (negative).

OBJECTIVE 6

The student should outline the initial management of inguinal lymphadenopathy.
A. The student should recognize that because most patients with penile cancer present with inguinal adenopathy due to infection rather than metastases, clinical assessment should be delayed 4–6 weeks while the patient is treated with antimicrobials.
B. Following antimicrobial therapy, the physical examination should be repeated and CT of the abdomen and pelvis performed.

OBJECTIVE 7

The student should outline management of inguinal lymphadenopathy that resolves after 4–6 weeks of antimicrobials.
A. The student should recognize that prophylactic ilioinguinal lymphadenectomy has not been demonstrated to enhance survival and is associated with considerable morbidity (particularly lower extremity lymphedema).
B. The student should recognize that sentinel lymph node biopsy is an option: not only are these nodes the first site of inguinal lymph node metastases, but relative to ilioinguinal lymphadenopathy the biopsy represents a relatively minor procedure. If the patient has bilaterally negative sentinel lymph node biopsies, he has approximately a 90% cure rate and should be followed with periodic examinations. If one or both sentinel nodes are positive, ilioinguinal lymph node dissection should be performed.

OBJECTIVE 8

The student should outline management of inguinal lymphadenopathy that persists after 4–6 weeks of antimicrobial therapy.
A. Ilioinguinal lymphadenectomy is the treatment of choice.
B. Sentinel lymph node biopsy remains an option as discussed in Objective 7.
C. Radiotherapy may be curative for inguinal lymph node metastases but has a lower cure rate than surgery does.

Achievement Level

Minimum Level of Achievement for Passing

The student should:
A. Be able to obtain the pertinent history and physical findings, make the provisional diagnosis of squamous cell carcinoma of the penis, and discuss the management of the primary tumor.
B. Recognize that therapeutic and not prophylactic ilioinguinal lymph node dissection should be performed.

Honors Level of Achievement

The student should:
A. Be able to differentiate the relative indications of partial versus total penectomy.
B. Recognize that sentinel lymph node biopsy is an acceptable method of evaluating the inguinal region in patients with penile cancer.